Chair Yoga for Weight Loss

Complete and Easy 28-Day Beginner, Intermediate, and Advanced Challenges to Lose Weight in Under 10-Minutes a Day

Robert H. Warren

Table of Contents

Introduction

As we age, losing weight and staying active can become increasingly challenging. Several factors contribute to this challenge, including slower metabolism, muscle loss, joint pain and stiffness, chronic health conditions, medication side effects, lifestyle changes, as well as mindset and motivation.

As I've gotten older, I've certainly come to face these challenges. I'd always enjoyed staying active throughout my life, and generally considered myself a physically fit person. However, there came a certain point when the changes in my body began to get in the way of certain physical activities.

This realization was hard on me. I didn't want to slow down, but I felt frustrated that I couldn't perform at the level I once did, and I eventually lost a lot of motivation to get up every day and do something active. On top of my diminishing motivation, I started to become busier and felt my priorities shifting. Work demands increased, family responsibilities grew, and time for exercise seemed to vanish.

I was feeling more sluggish and less confident; I started developing health issues; and I ultimately really missed the feeling of strength and vitality that came with being active. So, I set out on a journey to reclaim my health and vitality to ultimately improve the quality of my life. Through my research, I stumbled upon the ancient practice of yoga – a discipline known for its unbounded capacity to enhance mobility, strength, and mindfulness in those who regularly practice it. However, due to my lack of mobility, and the weight I had gained over the years, I found it particularly challenging to practice traditional yoga.

A friend of mine suggested that I explore chair yoga, a gentle and accessible practice modification suited to those with limited mobility, such as seniors like you and me. I decided it wouldn't hurt to try, so I went to a class with him. From the first session, I was hooked. It provided exactly what I needed. The low-impact workout still challenged me both physically and mentally and it was the perfect way to ease back into exercise without burning out or injuring myself.

As I continued with chair yoga, I noticed I was also sleeping better, feeling less stressed, and making healthier food choices. Slowly but surely, I started losing weight and regaining my confidence. Best of all, I could get out and do more of the things I loved.

In this book, you'll be introduced to the fundamentals of chair yoga and exercises that you can do in the comfort of your own home, based on poses that helped me get back into working out and progress into the physically fit person I am today.

You may feel skeptical about the benefits of chair yoga, and you're not alone. I was admittedly skeptical when I first heard about it, but once I committed to the practice, I was astonished at the transformative path it led me down—both physically and mentally.

Remember that you've already taken the first step: Deciding you want to make a change in your life.

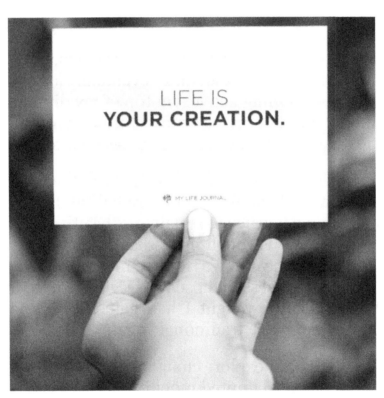

Chapter 1:

28-Day Weight Loss Challenge

Overview of Chair Yoga

Chair yoga is a gentler form of yoga that is practiced sitting on a chair or standing, using a chair for support. It offers a modified approach to traditional yoga poses, making it accessible to a wider range of people. Because yoga is traditionally practiced on a floor mat, it has various obstacles for certain individuals, including seniors, people with disabilities, pregnant women, or anyone who finds it challenging to practice on a mat. By incorporating a chair, chair yoga provides support and stability, making it easier to perform poses.

One of the great things about chair yoga is that it can be done anywhere. Whether you're at home, at work, or traveling, chair yoga is a convenient option if you have a busy schedule or don't have access to a yoga studio. Despite being practiced while seated, chair yoga helps improve flexibility, strength, and balance by engaging in a series of gentle stretches and movements that target different muscle groups. The gentle movements and stretches encourage blood flow, which can be beneficial, especially if you have circulation issues or a lifestyle that requires you to sit for long periods of time. Just like traditional yoga, chair yoga emphasizes breathwork and mindfulness, promoting relaxation and stress reduction. The mental element of chair yoga can be particularly beneficial for those dealing with issues such as anxiety or chronic pain.

Benefits of Chair Yoga for Weight Loss

Chair yoga offers a gentle yet effective way to improve fitness and overall health. It can help boost your metabolism, which is the rate at which your body burns calories. By engaging in gentle movements and stretches, chair yoga can stimulate the metabolism and help promote weight loss.

Yoga practices stand out among other exercise regimens because of their emphasis on holistic health. Incorporating mental elements in conjunction with chair yoga's physical elements promotes overall well-being. Mental health is closely tied to physical health, and improving one area will also help boost the other. For example, stress is directly correlated with weight gain. Chair yoga emphasizes deep breathing and relaxation, which can help reduce stress levels both at the immediate level and in the long term. High-stress levels can often lead to emotional eating, hormone changes that cause you to feel hungrier, poor-quality sleep, and decreased energy levels, all of which contribute to weight gain. Managing stress through chair yoga can help combat these symptoms and support your weight-loss efforts.

Through chair yoga, you will engage in gentle strength-building exercises that help tone your muscles. As you build muscle mass, your body replaces fat with muscle, and your body also becomes more efficient at burning calories, which can aid in weight loss. Chair yoga also helps improve flexibility, which can make it easier to engage in other forms of physical activity and lead a more active lifestyle. Being more flexible can also help prevent injuries during exercise, allowing you to maintain a consistent workout routine.

Practicing mindfulness during chair yoga will also help increase your self-awareness in other aspects of your daily life. Once you get more accustomed to mindfulness, it can help you become more aware of your eating habits. By paying attention to how and what you eat, you will be more likely to make healthier choices and avoid overeating. It also helps boost energy levels, making you feel more motivated to engage in an active lifestyle. With more sustained energy, you will likely find it easier to stick to a regular exercise routine and achieve your weight-loss goals.

Introduction to the 28-Day Challenges

The 28-day challenges have been specifically designed to ease you into your chair yoga practice, allowing you to gradually incorporate chair yoga into your routine and increase its intensity and complexity as you move from the beginner challenge to the intermediate to advanced challenge. Each week, you will be able to progress toward more and more challenging poses and build your experience with chair yoga to eventually be able to practice advanced level poses.

Before you begin with any of the 28-day challenges, you'll want to review all the poses outlined in its chapter. Once you feel familiar with the poses, look at the 28-day challenge for the particular level and stick with it for 28-days to fully benefit from it. I always recommend getting started with the beginner-level 28-day challenge before moving on to the intermediate and advanced challenges, regardless of your fitness level. Because yoga is a holistic practice, it's important to fully understand the guiding principles, like how to properly breathe as you move through the physical exercises, how to stay mindful throughout your routine, and the different elements of physicality that yoga targets (balance, mobility, strength, and flexibility).

The 28-day challenges are broken up into four unique weekly routines that are designed to gradually build in intensity and duration. In week 1 of each challenge, you will practice 3 poses per session, with each session lasting up to 10 minutes for a total of 3 sessions in the week. In week 2, you will practice 4 poses per session, with each session lasting up to 10 minutes, for a total of 4 sessions in the week. During weeks 3–4, you will practice 5 poses per session, with each session lasting up to 10 minutes, for a total of 5 sessions each week.

Key Takeaways

If you're new to chair yoga, it's beneficial to start with shorter sessions and gradually increase the duration and intensity as you become more comfortable. Always listen to your body and resist pushing yourself too hard. This is especially important when you're just starting because even if you already lead an active lifestyle, chair yoga will work areas that you may not be used to, such as certain muscle groups or elements like balance. Remember that everyone's body is different, so it's essential to pay attention to how you're feeling and modify poses as needed. If something doesn't feel right, don't force it. Instead, find a variation of the pose that works for you. Consistency is key to reaping the full benefits of chair yoga. This is where the 28-day challenge comes in to keep you motivated. As you progress through the challenge, you'll notice improvements in your flexibility, strength, and overall well-being, making your yoga routine feel more familiar and enjoyable.

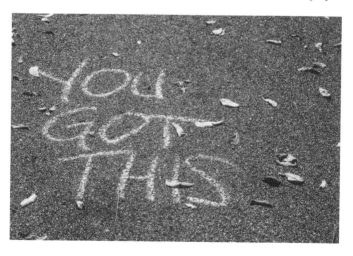

Chapter 2:

Getting Started

Preparing Your Space

Preparing a designated space for chair yoga is key to creating a conducive environment for your practice. First, you'll want to select a quiet, clutter-free space where you can focus and move without distractions. Make sure to remove any obstacles or furniture that could get in the way of your movements. This will allow you to move freely and safely throughout your sessions.

Next, you'll want to choose the chair you'll be using to practice. Ensure that your chair is stable and supportive. Avoid chairs with wheels or armrests that could hinder your movements or potentially be dangerous.

Before jumping in, double-check that your chair is placed on a stable, even surface and won't slip. Check that there is enough space around you to move your arms and legs without hitting anything.

Setting Realistic Goals

Taking the time to set goals for yourself is crucial for motivation and success. However, it is equally important to make sure that these goals challenge you while also staying realistic. If your goals are too far-fetched or not specific enough, they may result in disappointment and hinder your motivation to continue.

Instead of setting a vague goal like "I want to lose weight," try to get more specific about how much weight you want to lose and by when. For example, a specific goal could look like, "I want to lose five pounds in the next two months." Breaking down your overall goal into smaller, measurable milestones can also be a helpful way to track long-term goals. For instance, if you want to lose 50 pounds to hit your target weight, breaking down how many pounds you want to lose per month can help you see your progress and celebrate your journey.

It can be tempting to just focus on the number on the scale; however, it's often more helpful to instead set goals related to behavior changes. For example, you may set goals like "I will eat vegetables with every meal" or "I will do something physical every day."

Choose goals that fit with your lifestyle and are sustainable in the long term. You'll get a better sense of what realistic goals for you look like as you move through your weight loss journey. With that in mind, it's important to be flexible and willing to adjust your goals when needed. If you're not seeing the progress you'd hoped for with a certain goal, instead of giving yourself a hard time, simply reassess and make changes accordingly.

Tracking Progress

Tracking your progress can be a powerful way to stay motivated and see how far you've come. Keeping a journal is a great way to record the steps you're taking to reach your goals. It's also an active way to reflect on the changes you're making and seeing as a result of incorporating chair yoga into your routine. Write about how you felt before and after a session, any positive changes you're seeing in other areas of your life, like increased mindfulness or getting better quality sleep, and any insights that arose during sessions.

Keep track of your flexibility by measuring your range of motion in key poses. You can use a tape measure or simply note how far you can reach in each pose. You can also track your strength by paying attention to how certain poses feel and whether they become easier over time. At the end of every week, you can measure your flexibility and record it in a journal. This way, you can review your progress and make sure you're on track or adjust accordingly to stay on track.

Modifications for Comfort and Safety

Paying attention to how your body feels during each pose is essential to preventing injury during chair yoga practice. Modify or skip any poses that cause discomfort or pain. It's important to honor your body's limits and not push yourself beyond what feels comfortable.

If sitting upright in a chair is uncomfortable, you can place a cushion or folded towel behind your lower back for support. You can also sit on a cushion or yoga block to elevate your hips and reduce strain on your knees and back.

For poses that involve extending the legs, such as seated forward bends, you can bend your knees or keep your feet flat on the floor to reduce strain on your hamstrings and lower back.

If raising your arms overhead is challenging, you can modify certain poses by keeping your arms by your sides or resting your hands on your thighs.

To protect your neck, avoid excessive twisting or tilting. Keep your neck in a neutral position and only turn it as far as is comfortable. You can also support your head with your hands during seated twists.

Key Takeaways

Chair yoga's accessibility is one of the reasons why it is growing in popularity. Just about anyone can practice chair yoga from the comfort of their own home. However, because you're practicing in your home and not at a studio, you'll need to make sure to choose the right space for your chair yoga sessions. Choose a quiet, comfortable area with enough room to move around. Use a sturdy chair without wheels or armrests, and make sure you're placing the chair on a non-slip surface.

Before you begin, take some time to pinpoint the specific goals you're looking to achieve. These goals should be realistically achievable and align with your fitness level and health objectives. As you progress, make sure to set new goals to continue pushing yourself.

Aim for regular practice but remember to be kind to yourself. If you miss a day that you had planned for chair yoga practice, try to do your planned routine the following day. While the 28-day plan provides you with structure and guidance, it also gives you a bit of wiggle room for when you want to perform your routines.

Chapter 3:

Beginner Level Challenge

What to Expect

Now that you've learned about the 28-day challenges and what to do in preparation for the challenge, it's time to get started! In this chapter, you'll be introduced to 20 beginner-level chair yoga poses to ease you into the transformative practice of chair yoga and build your confidence. These poses are designed to improve flexibility, increase strength, and enhance overall well-being—all while accommodating your unique needs and physical limitations.

Each pose will be accompanied with step-by-step instructions on how to perform the exercises, and useful considerations to ensure safety and promote maximum benefit. You'll also be guided through proper breathing techniques for certain yoga exercises in order to get the most out of them.

Remember to review all of the poses first, making sure you understand their purpose, requirements, and sequences, before going through the 28-day beginner challenge. This way, you can move with intention when it comes time to put your practice into action.

As you go through the 28-day challenge, feel free to look back at the instructions of each of the poses you will be completing on a particular day to remind yourself of the exact steps you need to take to complete each pose properly and safely.

Beginner Poses for Arms

Up and Down Arms

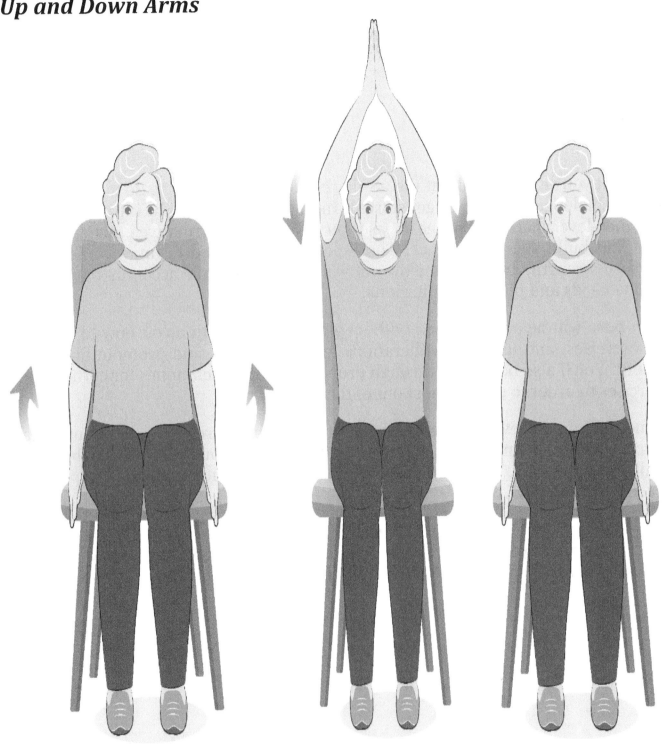

Set up:

- Place your chair in the area you've chosen to practice your chair yoga.

- Make sure that you have enough free space to reach your arms out to your sides and above your head while sitting in the chair without hitting anything.

Instructions:

- Sit comfortably in your chair with your arms resting by your sides.

- On an inhale, bring your arms out and up, reaching above your head to clasp your hands in a prayer position.

- Make sure to keep your back straight, shoulders relaxed, and head aligned with your spine.

- On an exhale, lower your arms back down by your sides.

- Repeat this motion ten times, allowing your breath to guide your movements.

- On the last exhale, lower your palms to rest on your thighs to come out of the exercise.

Key considerations:

- Your movements during this exercise should be fluid and loose.

- Remember to let your breathing guide your motions instead of the other way around. This will allow you to move at a slower, more natural pace and prevent you from going through the motions too quickly.

- Instead of keeping your arms straight and rigid, maintain a slight bend at your elbows to prevent them from locking. You should feel your arms start to warm up with this gentle exercise.

Cactus Pose

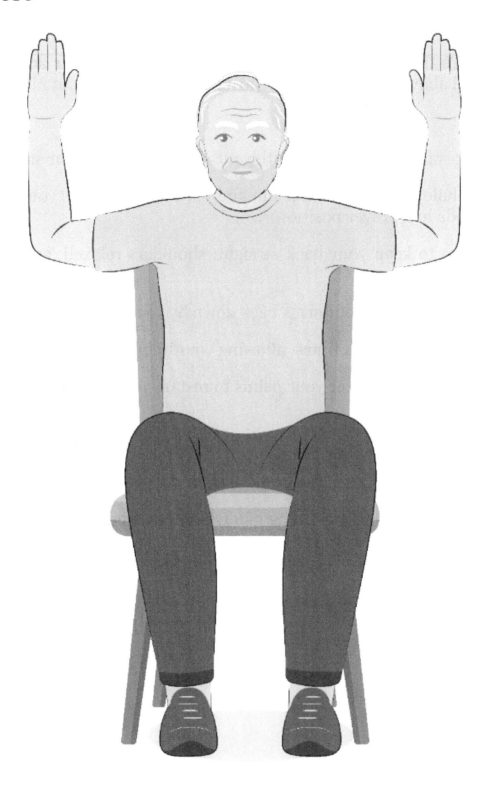

Set up:

- Place your chair in your designated chair yoga space.

- Check that you have enough free space around the chair to move your arms freely in all directions while seated.

Instructions:

- Sit comfortably in your chair with your palms resting on your thighs.

- On an inhale, raise your arms out to your sides so that they are parallel to the floor.

- On an exhale, bend your arms at the elbows so that your arms are at a 90-degree angle, with your fingertips pointing toward the ceiling and your palms facing forward.

- Feel your chest expand with every inhale, and your arm muscles engage with every exhale.

- Do not slouch or lean forward or backward as you hold this pose to avoid any unnecessary strain on your back.

- Hold this position for five deep breaths.

- On the final exhale, bring your arms down, resting your palms on your thighs to completely release from the pose.

- Repeat this exercise once through.

Key considerations:

- When holding the cactus pose, make sure that your upper arms are parallel with the floor at shoulder height. Your forearms should be perpendicular to the upper arms, with your hands in line with your elbows.

- Remember to keep your arm muscles engaged while holding this pose to maintain proper form.

Arm Rotations

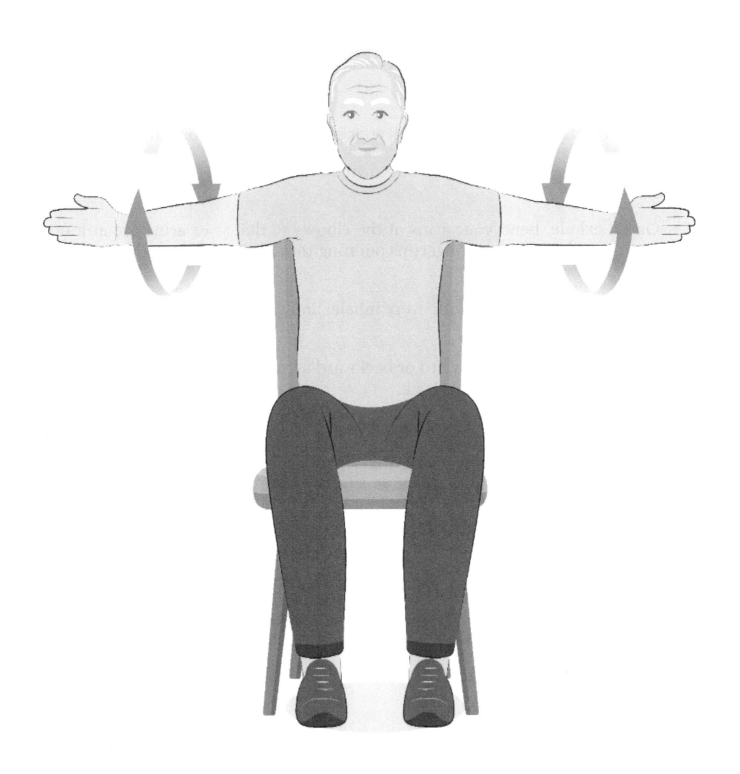

Set up:

- Place your chair in your designated chair yoga space, and make sure there's enough room around you to extend your arms in all directions without hitting anything.

Instructions:

- Sit comfortably in your chair.

- On an inhale, raise your arms out to your sides so that they are parallel to the floor.

- Keep your fingertips outstretched.

- Exhale and begin to move your arms in a circular motion, like you're drawing large circles with your fingertips.

- Maintain this motion for five deep breaths, then slowly come to a stop, and on an exhale, bring your arms back down to rest.

- On an inhale, raise your arms out to your sides again and begin to move them in circulation motion in the opposite direction.

- Draw your circles in this direction for five more deep breaths.

- Slowly bring your arms to a stop, and on an exhale, bring your arms back down to rest.

- Repeat this exercise once through.

Key considerations:

- Make sure you remember to breathe throughout this exercise and that your motions are slow and controlled to maintain proper form.

- Maintain a slight bend at the elbows to ensure you're not locking your joints.

- Engage your arm muscles and relax your shoulders so that you're not carrying unnecessary tension.

Sun Breaths

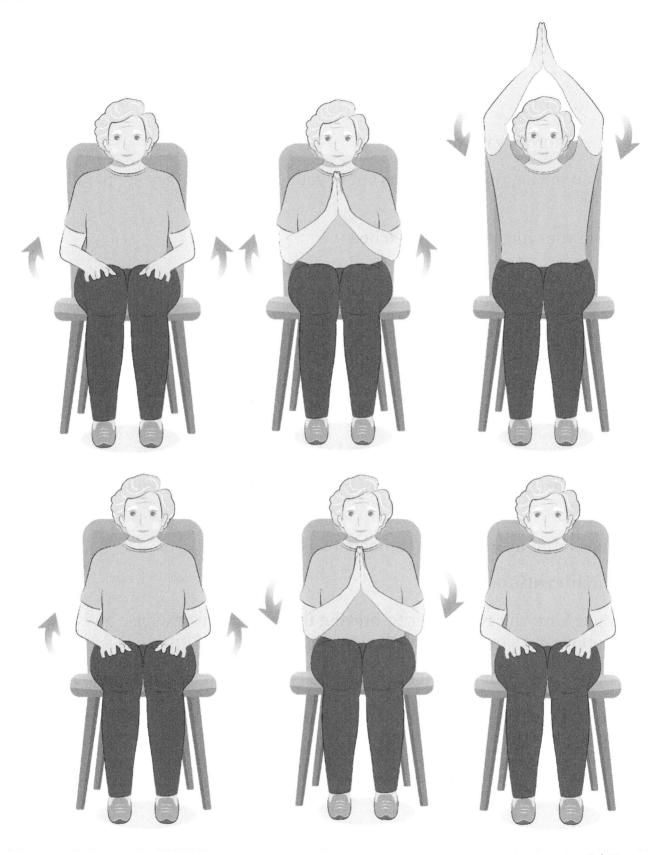

Set up:

- Place your chair in the space you're using for your chair yoga practice.

- Check to see if you're able to move your arms freely in all directions while seated without bumping into anything.

Instructions:

- Sit comfortably in your chair with your palms resting on your thighs.

- On an inhale, bring your palms together in front of your heart in a prayer pose.

- Exhale while holding this position.

- Inhale and slowly bring your arms out and up above your head, reaching your fingertips toward the ceiling.

- Exhale and slowly lower your arms out and down, maintaining the stretch in your arms.

- Inhale and bring your palms together in front of your heart once again.

- Lower your palms to your thighs to come out of this exercise.

- Repeat this sequence five times, paying attention to your breath and letting it guide your movements.

Key considerations:

- Your movements during this exercise should be fluid. Allowing your breath to guide you will help you with this.

- Engage your arm muscles to keep your movements slow and controlled.

Beginner Poses for the Neck and Shoulders

Head Tilt

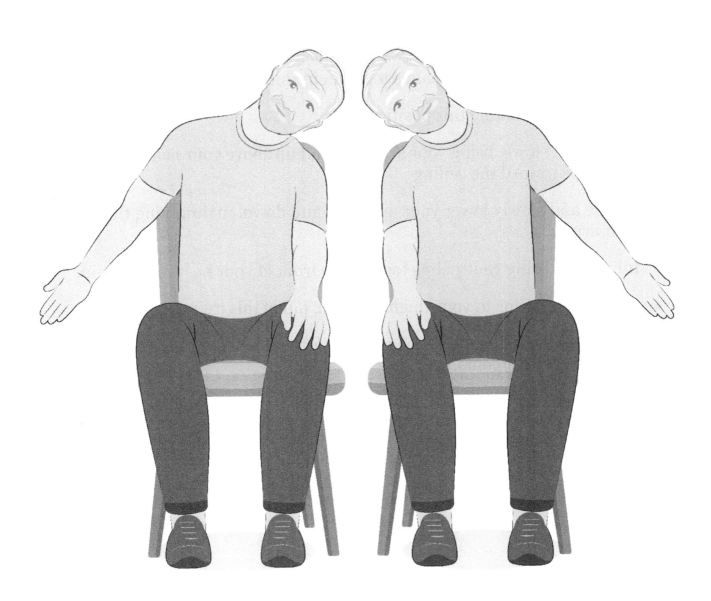

Set up:

- Place your chair in your designated chair yoga space, and make sure there's enough room around you to extend your arms in all directions without hitting anything.

Instructions:

- Sit comfortably in your chair with your palms resting on your thighs.

- Slowly raise your right arm a little bit away from your body.

- Next, gently tilt your head to the left.

- The position of your right arm should be in line with your head position, so if you were to draw a line from the top of your head to your fingertips, it would be straight.

- Bring your right arm gently back behind your body.

- Your palm should be facing forward.

- Hold this position for three deep breaths, feeling a gentle stretch on the right side of your neck, your right shoulder, and your right arm.

- Slowly release, bringing your head back to the center and your arm back in its initial resting position to come out of the pose.

- Repeat this sequence once more on the other side.

Key considerations:

- Don't force your head to tilt in one direction more than is comfortable.

- You should feel a nice stretch in your neck, shoulders, and arms, but nothing that causes pain or discomfort.

Shoulder Rolls

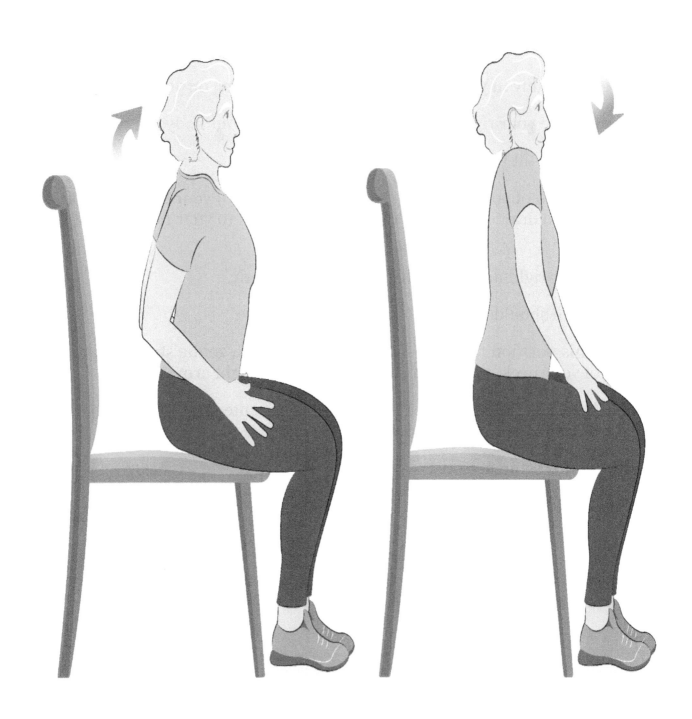

Set up:

- Place your chair in your designated chair yoga space, and make sure there's enough room around you to extend your arms in all directions without hitting anything.

Instructions:

- Sit comfortably on your chair, letting your arms hang down by your sides.

- Take a few deep breaths and slide forward slightly to make a gap between your back and the backrest of the chair.

- On an inhale, slowly bring your shoulders back and then up toward your ears in a circular, forward-facing motion.

- As you exhale, continue circling your shoulders in this direction, moving them forward and then down.

- Repeat this sequence for five deep breaths making five forward-facing circles.

- At the end of the fifth rotation, slow to a stop before changing directions and repeating the process, moving the opposite way for five full breaths, making five circles in backward-facing direction.

- At the end of this routine, let your shoulders drop down and back, paying attention to how loose and tension-free your shoulders feel as you come out of this exercise.

- Repeat once through.

Key considerations:

- Allow your breath to guide your motions. Make sure that you are taking full, deep breaths. This will ensure that your motions are slow and controlled.

- Your movements should be fluid and led by your shoulders. The rest of your body should be relaxed and still.

- If you feel that you're holding tension in any part of your body, such as your neck, gently pause your movements to release that tension, and then continue with the exercise.

Eagle Arms

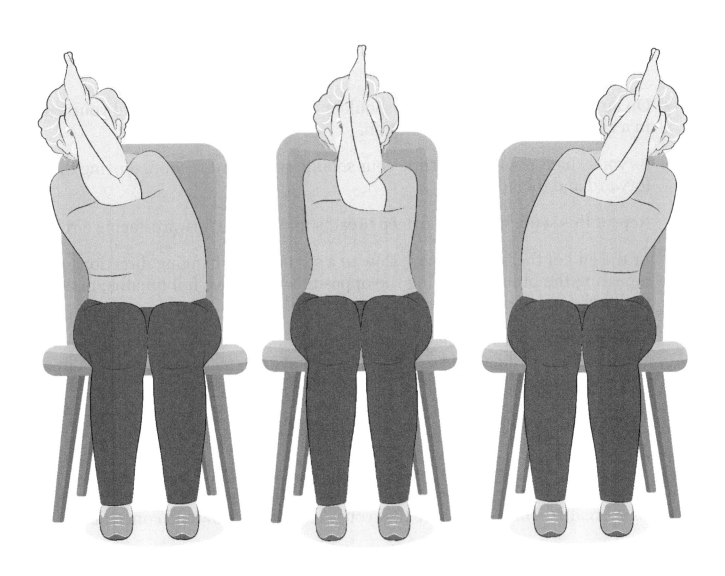

Set up:

- Place your chair in your designated chair yoga space, and make sure that you have enough room to move freely without hitting anything.

Instructions:

- Sit comfortably in your chair and bring your arms out in front of you.

- Bend your elbows upwards so that your arms are at a 90-degree angle, with your fingers pointing toward the ceiling.

- Place your right arm over your left arm so that the area just above your right elbow is resting in the crook of your left elbow.

- Gently rotate your forearms so that you can bring your palms together.

- Holding this position, inhale and slowly raise your elbows.

- As you exhale, slowly lower them back slightly to feel a light stretch between your shoulder blades.

- Repeat this motion for four deep breaths, allowing your breath to guide your movements before slowly coming back to the center.

- From here, inhale and tilt your eagle arms to your right, allowing your upper body to move with your arms. Exhale and return to the center.

- On your next inhale, repeat this on your left side.

- Repeat this sequence for four full breaths before coming back to the center.

- To come out of the pose, slowly release your arms from their position, and then repeat the same sequence once more with your left arm over your right.

Key considerations:

- If you're unable to position your arms in the eagle arms position, you can modify this pose by simply bringing your forearms together and connecting your elbows and palms.

- Make sure to keep a straight back and keep your shoulders relaxed as you practice this pose to avoid any unnecessary strain.

Elbow Rotations

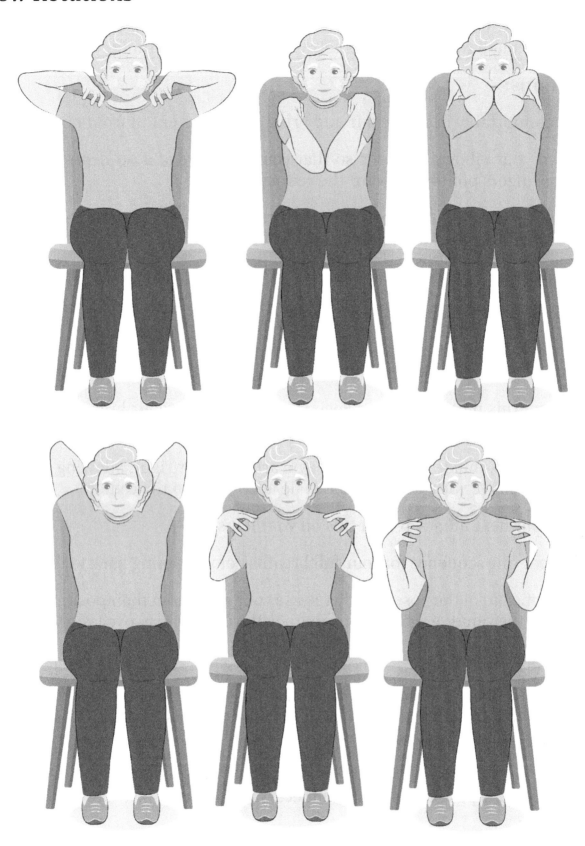

Set up:

- Place your chair in your designated chair yoga space, and make sure there's enough room around you to extend your arms in all directions without hitting anything.

Instructions:

- Sit comfortably in your chair and bring your fingertips up to touch their respective shoulders.

- On an inhale, bring your elbows forward and toward each other until they touch.

- You should feel a light stretch between your shoulder blades.

- Next, bring your elbows up and over your head, reaching them up toward the ceiling.

- Exhale and bring your elbows back and then down, feeling your chest open up.

- Once they come back down, your shoulders should feel completely relaxed as you release any remaining tension.

- Slowly tilt your head up and down and then side to side, releasing any remaining tension in your neck and feeling it loosen up.

- Repeat the elbow circles four more times, remembering to let your breath guide your fluid motions.

- To release from this pose, bring your hands down from your shoulders and let your palms rest on your thighs.

- Repeat in the opposite direction for five elbow rotations.

Key considerations:

- Remember to work through these motions slowly. Letting your breath guide your movements will help you with this.

- Lead your movements with your elbows. This will help you get rid of any tension in your shoulders, upper back, and neck.

Beginner Poses for Chest and Back

Spinal Twist

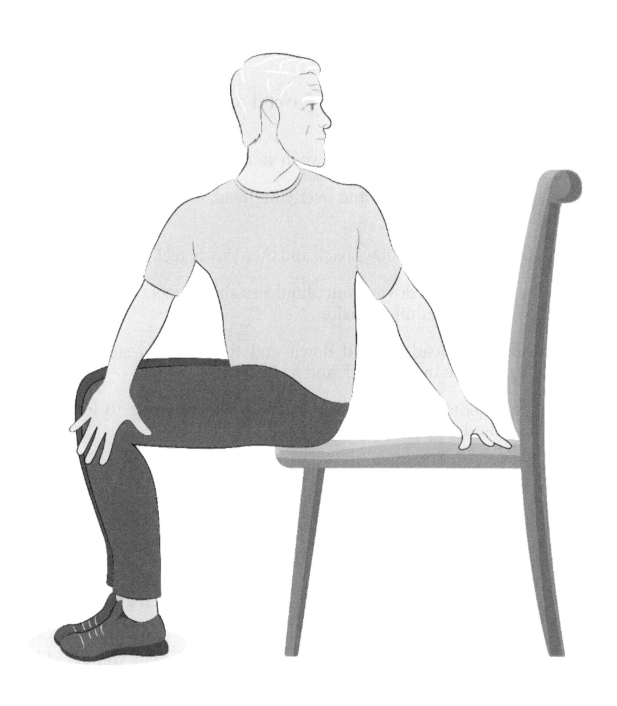

Set up:

- Set your chair in your designated space for chair yoga.

- Check that you have sufficient room to comfortably move around.

Instructions:

- Sit comfortably in your chair, and scoot forward a bit so that you are seated more toward the edge of your chair.

- Place your right arm on the outer side of your left knee. Feel free to grab your knee if you find it difficult to keep your arm in this position.

- On an inhale, twist your torso toward the left side and bring your left arm toward the back of your chair, with your palm resting where the back and seat of the chair meet.

- Gently press down your left hand on the seat and press down your right hand against your left knee to get a deeper stretch.

- To release from this pose, slowly release your arms, bringing them down to rest at your sides.

- Slowly untwist your torso back to a neutral seated position. Let your palms rest on your thighs.

- On an inhale, twist in the opposite direction, and repeat the steps on your right side.

- Repeat this sequence six times.

Key considerations:

- Make sure to move into and out of the twists slowly.

- Breathing deeply into each twist will help control the pace of your movements.

- Resist forcing the twist; instead, twist as far as feels comfortable.

- Engage your core and sit tall in your chair to ensure you are maintaining proper posture.

Cat/Cow

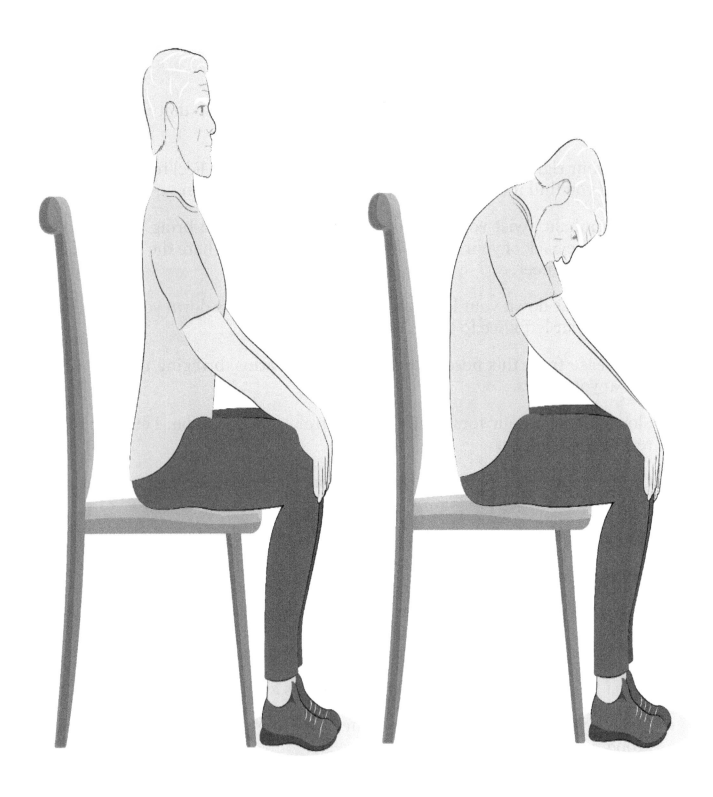

Set up:

- Place your chair in your designated chair yoga space, and make sure there's enough room around you to extend your arms in all directions without hitting anything.

Instructions:

- Sit comfortably on your chair with your palms resting on your thighs.

- Scoot down a bit so that you're seated more toward the edge of your seat.

- On an inhale, slowly arch your spine, bringing your shoulders and head back.

- Hold here for a moment, feeling your chest opening up. This is the cow pose.

- On an exhale, slowly round your back by moving your shoulders forward and your head down while pulling your navel back toward your spine.

- You should feel a nice stretch in your upper back. This is the cat pose.

- Hold here for a moment and release all the tension in your neck, letting your head hang forward.

- Repeat the cow and cat poses five times, allowing your breath to guide you into each pose.

- To come out of this exercise, slowly move from the cat pose back to a neutral seated position by uncurling your back, shoulders, and head on an inhale.

Key considerations:

- While in the cat pose, instead of forcing your chin to your chest, simply release any tension in your neck to let your head drop down.

- Similarly, while in the cow pose, don't force your head back; instead, think about lengthening your neck and sending your gaze however far upwards is comfortable.

- Make sure your shoulders are always dropped down instead of bunched up by your ears to avoid creating any tension in your shoulders and neck.

Two Chair Forward Fold

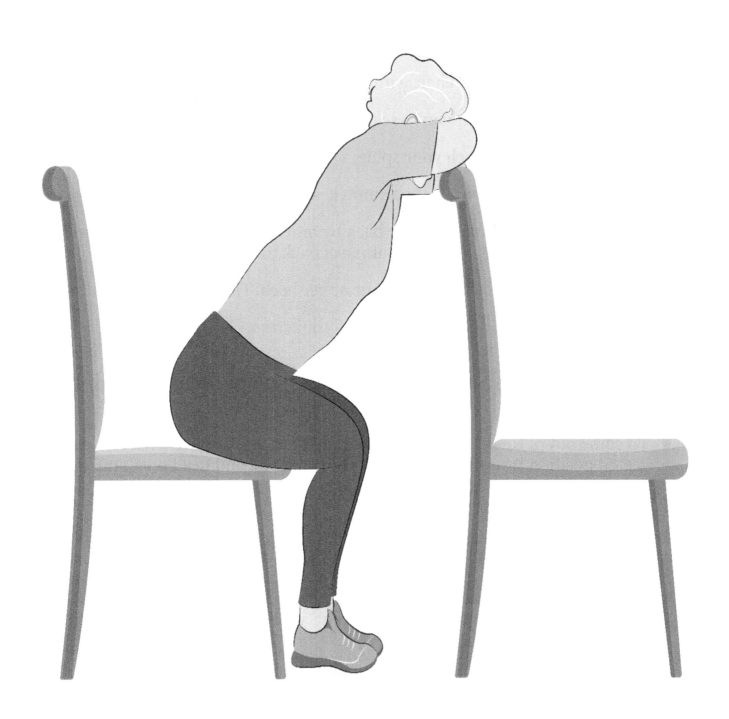

Set up:

- Bring two chairs to an open, comfortable area to practice chair yoga.

- Place one chair in front of the other so that you are able to sit on one chair and reach the back of the chair in front of you.

Instructions:

- Sit comfortably on the back chair and take a few deep breaths.

- On an exhale, bring your torso forward, hinging at the hips.

- Rest your arms on the other chair's back, folding one arm over the other.

- Rest your head on your folded arms.

- Inhale and drop your shoulders down and back, relaxing your arms and neck completely.

- Exhale and feel yourself drop deeper into the position as your body completely relaxes.

- Remain in this position for ten deep breaths.

- To release, slowly raise your torso upright on an inhale. Bring your palms down to your thighs.

- Repeat twice through, taking five deep breaths in between each repetition.

Key considerations:

- You can place the front chair against a wall to prevent any potential slipping of the chair when you put your upper body weight on it.

- Engage your core to ensure that your back is straight instead of arched or hunched and that you're breathing properly.

Cobra Pose

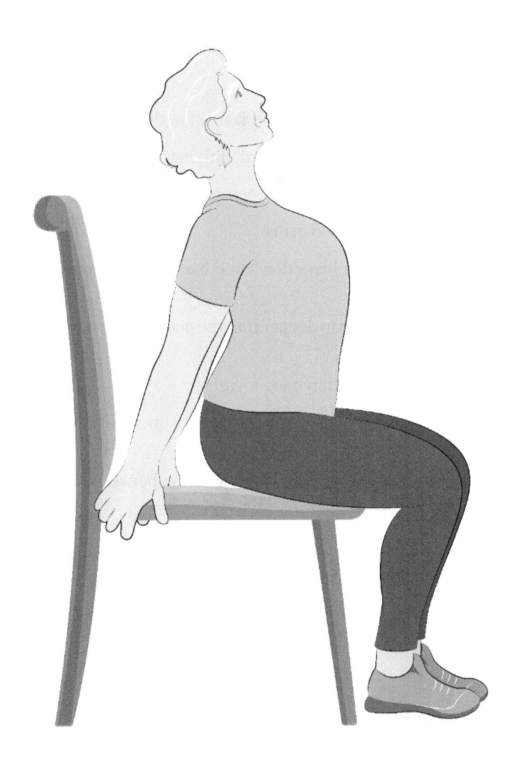

Set up:

- Bring your chair to your designated chair yoga space, and double-check that there are no objects in the vicinity that may get in the way of your movements.

Instructions:

- Sit comfortably at the edge of your chair.

- Reach your hands behind you, grabbing the area of the chair where the seat and back meet on either side.

- Inhale and raise your chest while you stretch your neck back and bring your gaze to the ceiling.

- Drop your shoulders down and back.

- Exhale and feel your chest expand further.

- Hold this pose for five deep breaths.

- To come out of the pose, slowly bring your head, then shoulders, then upper back to center as you straighten your spine.

- Release your hands from the chair and gently bring them forward to rest on your thighs.

- Repeat this exercise once through.

Key considerations:

- When arching your neck, instead of dropping your head back, think about lengthening the neck and sending your gaze upward.

- During this pose, it can be tempting to force the arch in your back; instead of doing so, focus on expanding your chest and relaxing your neck and shoulders. This will allow you to feel a nice stretch in your chest area and help release any tension you may be carrying in your upper body.

Beginner Poses for Abs

Marches

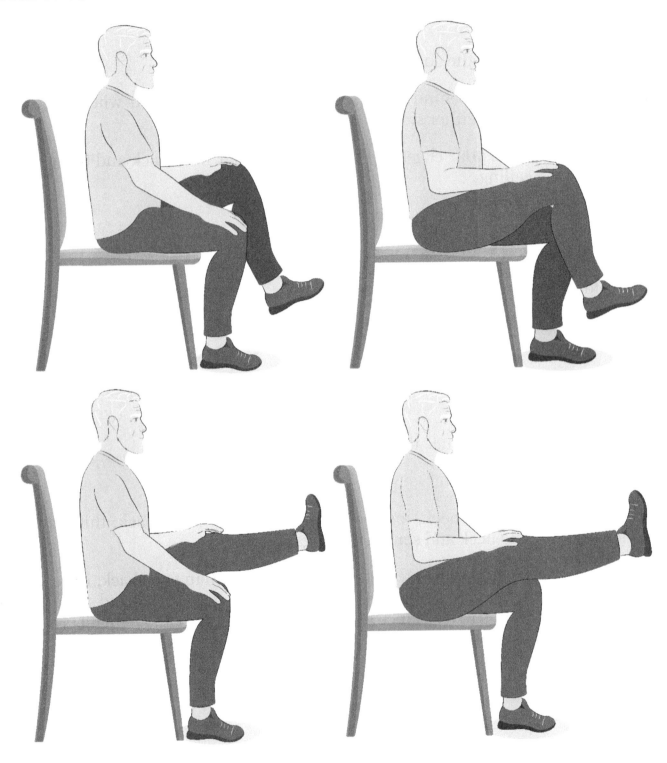

Set up:

- Bring your chair to a comfortable and accessible area to practice chair yoga freely.

Instructions:

- Sit comfortably in your chair with your palms resting on your thighs.

- Engage your core and bring your left leg up off the floor and then place it back down.

- Then bring your right leg up off the floor and then place it back down.

- Repeat this marching motion ten times.

- Next, bring your left leg up into a marching position and hold it up.

- On an inhale, extend your leg, straightening your left leg in the air.

- Exhale, hinge at the knee to bring your leg back to a marching position, and then lower your foot back to the floor.

- Repeat the march with the added extension with the right leg and then alternate between the two legs for 10 repetitions.

- To come out of this exercise, slow your legs to a stop, resting both feet flat on the floor.

Key considerations:

- When extending your legs, make sure to always maintain a slight bend at the knee to avoid overextending or locking the knees.

- Bring your awareness to your core during this exercise, making sure to keep your abdominal muscles engaged.

- Remember to keep breathing throughout this pose and let your breathing guide your marches.

Foot Hover

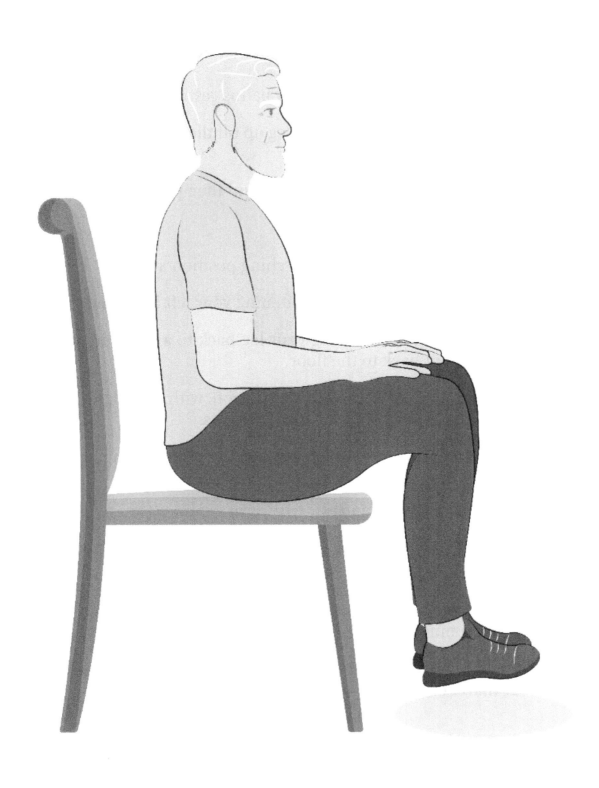

Set up:

- Place your chair in your designated area to practice chair yoga, making sure that you have sufficient room for optimal comfort.

Instructions:

- Sit comfortably in your chair with your palms resting on your thighs.

- Engage your core and lift your feet off the floor a couple of inches.

- If you are finding it hard to lift your feet up, try holding the sides of the chair with your hands, and pressing your hands into the chair as you lift your feet off of the floor.

- Hold this position for about 30 seconds, remembering to breathe throughout.

- To come out of this pose, gently bring both legs to a 90-degree angle as you lower your feet to rest flat on the floor.

- Repeat this exercise once through.

- If you want to make this exercise more challenging, you can add leg extensions.

- While your feet are hovering above the floor, slowly extend one leg, then bring it back to its original bent hover position, then repeat with the other leg.

- To make it even more challenging, instead of extending one leg at a time, try extending both legs at the same time.

Key considerations:

- With many abdominal exercises, people tend to hold their breath or restrict their breathing. This is especially true when you are in a position that works your abs. To make sure that you're breathing properly, bring your attention to your rib cage. As you inhale, you should be able to feel and see your rib cage expanding. As you exhale, you should feel and see it contract.

- With shallow breathing, tension is often held in the shoulders. Checking that your shoulders are relaxed and not held up toward your ears will also help ensure that you're practicing proper deep breathing as you move through this exercise.

Core Twists

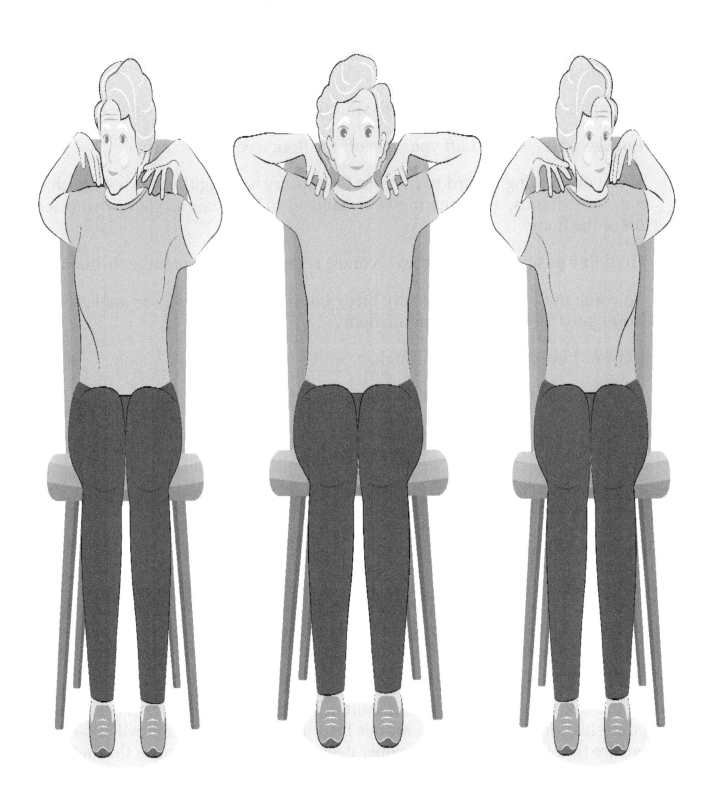

Set up:

- Place your chair in your designated chair yoga area, checking that the environment is not restrictive to your movement while seated in the chair.

Instructions:

- Sit comfortably in your chair.

- Inhale and bring your fingertips up to your shoulders with your elbows pointing out toward your sides and your chest wide.

- Take a few deep breaths to settle into this position.

- Make sure to keep your back straight and your shoulders relaxed.

- Next, engage your core and begin to twist your torso to the right side.

- Exhale and bring your torso back to the center.

- Next, engage your core again and twist your torso to the left side.

- Exhale again and bring your torso back to the center.

- Keep twisting for about 30 seconds.

- Keep your movement fluid from one side to the other and slowly focus on increasing your range of motion.

- To come out of this exercise, gently slow your torso to a stop and release your arms back down. Rest your palms on your thighs.

- Repeat this exercise once through.

Key considerations:

- While twisting, choose a pace that feels comfortable to you. If going slower feels better, stick with that. If you want to pick the pace up a bit, you can do so, but make sure that you aren't feeling any discomfort in your spine.

- If you feel any discomfort in your back, stop immediately and make sure your back is warmed up properly by repeating small twisting movements before trying this pose again.

Crunches

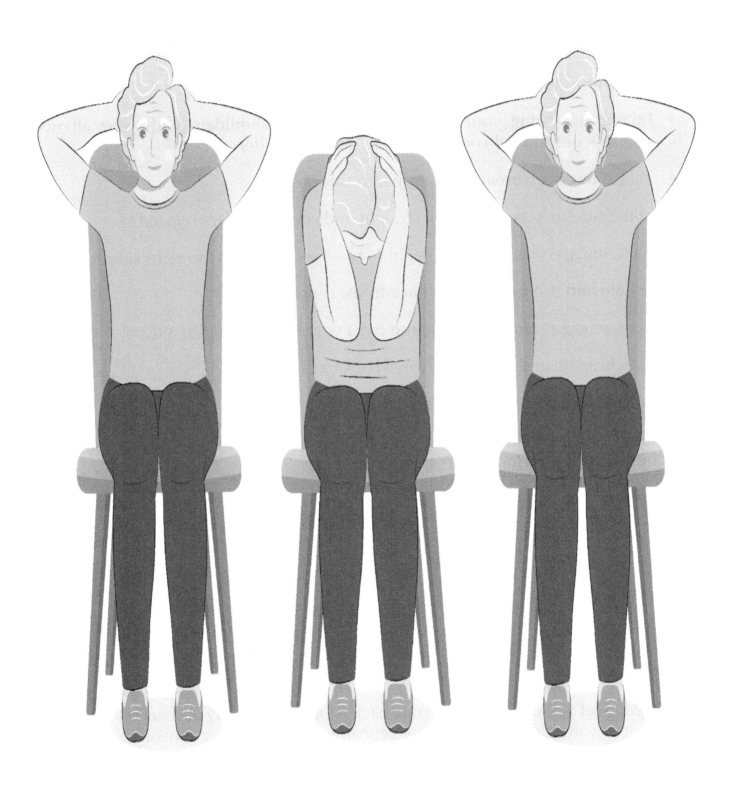

Set up:

- Bring your chair to a comfortable space to practice chair yoga, free from distractions.

Instructions:

- Sit comfortably in your chair.

- Inhale and bring your arms up to interlace your fingers behind your head.

- Feel your chest expand as you send your elbows out from your body.

- Engage your core, take a deep breath, and on the exhale, slowly round your back to bring your head down closer toward your thighs.

- Bring your elbows inwards and down toward your thighs.

- Inhale and using your core muscles, slowly rise back up to a seated position, bringing up your head and elbows to their first position.

- Repeat this sequence six times.

- After your last repetition, release your fingers from their interlaced position and slowly bring your palms down to rest on your thighs to come out of this exercise.

Key considerations:

- When you're moving into the crunch position, instead of forcing your chin into your chest, allow your head to drop however far is comfortable for you while supporting an extended neck with your interlaced fingers.

- Make sure you're actively engaging your core throughout this exercise to prevent putting strain on your back.

- Also, check to see if you are carrying tension on your shoulders. If you feel that you are, drop them down and back so that they are relaxed.

Beginner Poses for Legs

Chair Pigeon

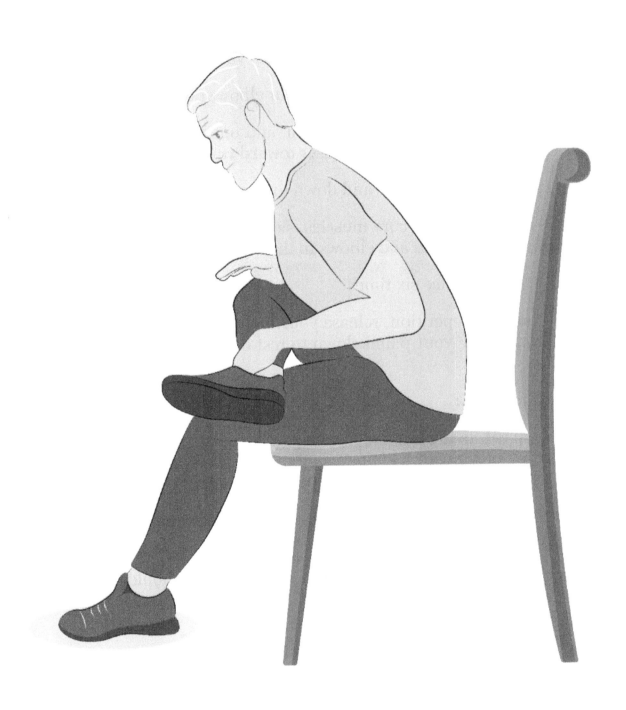

Set up:

- Bring your chair to a comfortable area to practice chair yoga, making sure there are no objects directly around the chair that would get in the way of your movement.

Instructions:

- Sit comfortably in your chair and bring your right foot up and over your left thigh so that your ankle is resting comfortably on the thigh.

- Place your right hand on your right knee and left hand on your right ankle and gently press them down.

- Make sure to keep your right ankle and knee parallel to the floor, with your knee pointing out to the right side.

- Hold this position, keeping your posture straight, for five deep breaths.

- Next, to deepen the stretch, slowly bend your torso forward, hinging at the hips until you feel your desired stretch level.

- Hold for another five deep breaths.

- Lift your torso back up to the starting position and then bring your right foot back to the floor. Bring your palms to your thighs.

- Repeat this sequence once more with your left leg.

Key considerations:

- When placing the ankle onto the thigh, check to see that your ankle is in line with its respective knee. This will help protect your knee by preventing any unnecessary strain and discomfort.

- If you're leaning forward to deepen the stretch, remember to maintain a straight, tall back. It's tempting to hunch the back a bit while deepening the stretch because it feels like you're moving further into the stretch, but if your back is rounded, you won't actually enhance the stretch. Think about lengthening the spine, keeping each vertebra in line up to the neck, and hinging at the hips.

Flexing Foot

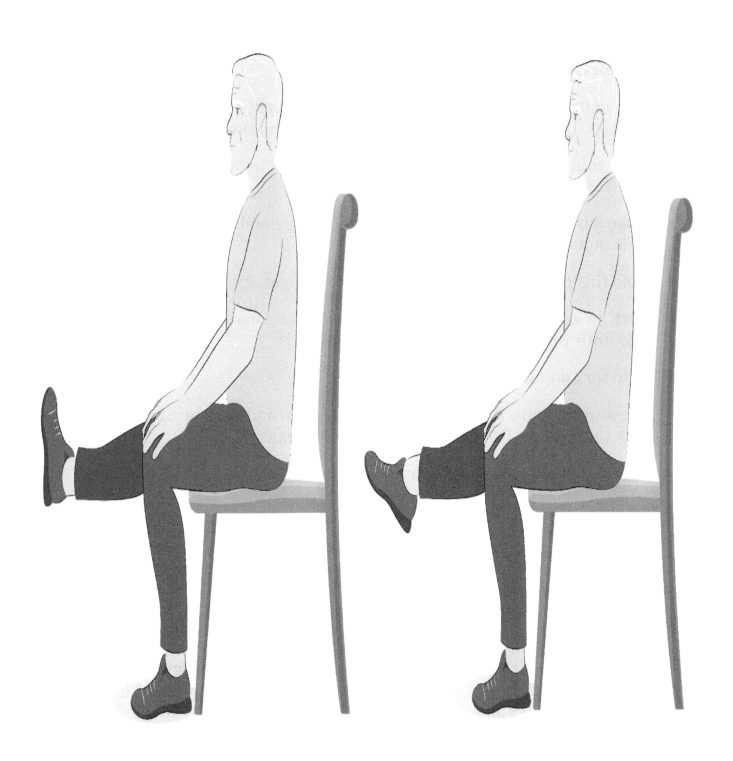

Set up:

- Bring your chair to your designated chair yoga space, and make sure that you have enough room to fully extend your legs while seated without bumping into anything.

Instructions:

- Sit comfortably in your chair with your palms resting on your thighs.

- On an inhale, raise your right leg so that it's extended straight in front of you.

- If you find this challenging, you can just lift your foot a few inches off of the floor.

- Feel free to grab the sides of the chair and press down into the seat of the chair to help you raise your leg.

- Next, flex your raised foot so that your toes are pointed toward the ceiling.

- Then, extend your foot so that your toes are pointed.

- Continue this pattern 10 times, alternating between flexing and pointing your foot and remembering to breathe throughout.

- After the last rep, lower your right foot back to rest on the floor and take a couple of deep breaths to relax.

- Repeat this sequence once more with your left foot.

Key considerations:

- Move at a pace that feels comfortable for you while feeling the stretch in the flexed and extended positions.

- Maintain a slight bend in the knee while working through this exercise to prevent overextending or locking the knee.

Tree Pose

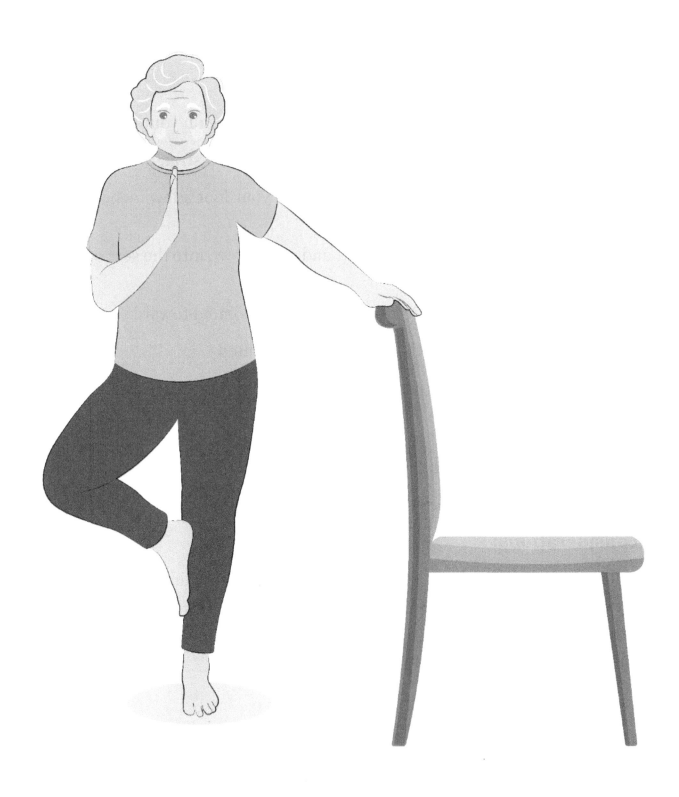

Set up:

- Bring your chair to a comfortable, open area. Make sure you have room to stand and move behind the chair.

Instructions:

- Come around to the back of your chair and stand on the right of the chair.

- Place your left hand on the back of the chair for stability.

- Take a few deep breaths in this standing position and feel the connection between the soles of your feet and the floor.

- Inhale and slowly bring your weight to your left foot and raise your right foot to place your right sole on the inside of your left calf or ankle. Exhale.

- Inhale and bring your right hand up to your heart, straightening the palm so that your hand is perpendicular to your chest with your fingers pointing toward the ceiling.

- Hold this pose for five deep breaths.

- To come out of the pose, slowly slide your raised foot down to the floor, lower your raised hand down to your side, and bring your hand on the chair down to your side as well.

- Next, turn around so that the chair is on your left side and repeat the sequence once more on this side.

Key considerations:

- Make sure you're standing tall with an aligned posture to maintain balance during this exercise. If you want to increase the difficulty, gradually loosen your grip on the chair, maintaining a lighter connection with the chair.

- Make sure to maintain a slight bend on your standing knee to ensure you aren't locking or overextending the joint.

Quad Lifts

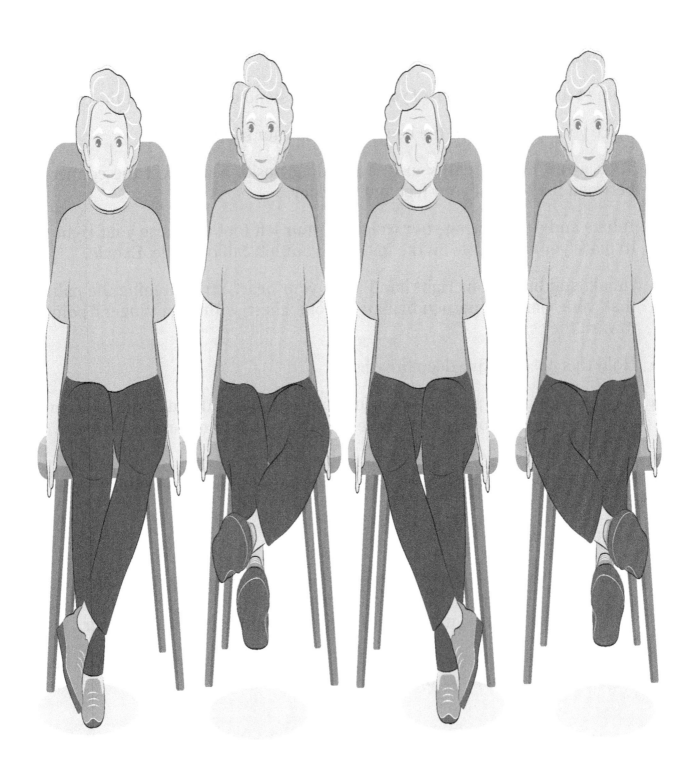

Set up:

- Bring your chair to a quiet, open space. Make sure that you have enough room to comfortably extend your legs while seated.

Instructions:

- Sit comfortably in your chair with your palms resting on your thighs.

- Bring your left foot over your right so that the ankle is resting on the shin of your right leg.

- Allow the weight of your left leg to rest on your right leg.

- Using your right leg, lift both legs by extending your right leg.

- Hold here for a couple of seconds before slowly lowering your right foot back down.

- If you are struggling to lift your feet up, grab the sides of your chair and press your hand into the chair to help you lift your legs.

- Repeat this ten times, remembering to breathe throughout, and then repeat the sequence ten times on the other side.

- To come out of this exercise, slowly lower the foot of your working leg down to the floor and bring the foot of the crossed leg down to the floor as well.

Key considerations:

- When lifting with the right leg, disengage the left leg completely, allowing its weight to be carried by the right leg and vice versa.

- When extending the working leg, make sure to maintain a slight bend at the knee at all times to avoid overextending the knee.

- Engaging your core will also help you maintain proper posture and form throughout this exercise.

Weekly Routine

Week 1

Day 1

- Begin with **Up and Down Arms** (page 10) for 10 repetitions.

- Bring your arms back down to neutral, letting your palms rest on your thighs. Take a few deep breaths here, letting yourself rest for about 15 seconds before moving into **Cat/Cow** (page 28) for five repetitions.

- Take a few deep breaths in a neutral seated position as you rest for about 15 seconds. Move into **Quad Lifts** (page 48) and repeat for 10 repetitions.

Day 2

- Begin with **Arm Rotations** (page 14) in one direction for five deep breaths and then in the opposite direction for five deep breaths.

- Bring your arms down to neutral and take a few deep breaths, resting for 15 seconds. Move into the **Eagle Arms** pose (page 22), going through the exercise once with the right arm over the left and then once more with the left arm over the right.

- Untwist, and let your palms rest on your thighs. Rest for 15 seconds. Move into the **Marches** exercise (page 38), going through the basic exercise 10 times and then through the exercise with the added leg extensions 10 times.

Day 3

- Begin with **Core Twists** (page 38) for about 30 seconds.

- Return to neutral, take a few deep breaths as you rest for 15 seconds, and then move into **Chair Pigeon** (page 42) for five deep breaths per side.

- Return to neutral, take a few deep breaths as you rest for 15 seconds, and finish out your session with **Sun Breaths** (page 16), performing five repetitions.

Week 2

Day 1

- Begin your session by moving through the **Cactus Pose** exercise (page 12). Hold the pose for five deep breaths, release, then perform one more repetition of the exercise. Return to a neutral seated position, and rest for about 10 seconds as you take a few deep breaths.

- Move into **Shoulder Rolls** (page 20), performing the exercise for five rotations moving in one direction, followed by five rotations moving in the opposite direction.

- Come back to neutral, take a few deep breaths as you rest for 10 seconds, and then move into **Two Chair Forward Fold** (page 30), performing the exercise for four repetitions.

- Return to neutral, and take a few deep breaths, resting for 10 seconds. Move into the **Flexing Foot** exercise (page 44) 10 times on your right foot and then 10 times on your left foot.

Day 2

- Begin your session with six repetitions of the **Spinal Twist** exercise (page 26). Scoot back in your chair and return to a neutral sitting position.

- Take a few deep breaths as you rest for 10 seconds, and then move into the **Foot Hover** exercise (page 36) for two repetitions for a total of about one minute. Rest for 10 seconds.

- Come to a standing position behind your chair, and move into **Tree Pose** (page 46), performing the exercise once through on both legs.

- Return to sitting, take a few deep breaths as you rest for about 10 seconds, and finish out your session with the **Head Tilt** (page 18), going through the exercise for three deep breaths per side.

Day 3

- Begin with **Elbow Rotations** (page 24), moving through the full exercise for five reps. Bring your arms back down to neutral and take a few deep breaths, resting for 10 seconds. Perform one more set of five reps, then come back to neutral, and rest for 10 more seconds.

- Move into **Cobra Pose** (page 32) and hold here for five deep breaths before returning to neutral.

- Rest for 10 seconds. Move into **Crunches** (page 40), performing six repetitions.

- Return to neutral and take a few deep breaths, resting for 10 seconds, before closing out your session with five **Sun Breaths** (page 16).

Day 4

- Begin by moving through the **Cactus Pose** exercise (page 12). Hold the pose for five deep breaths, release, then perform one more repetition of the exercise. Come back to neutral, resting for 10 seconds as you take deep, grounding breaths.

- Move into **Shoulder Rolls** (page 20), performing five forward rotations followed by five backward rotations.

- Return to neutral, rest for 10 seconds, and move into **Quad Lifts** (page 48), performing 10 repetitions per leg.

- Return to neutral and take a few deep breaths, resting for 10 seconds. Finish out with **Cat/Cow** (page 28), performing five repetitions.

Week 3

Day 1

- Begin with **Marches** (page 34), performing 10 repetitions of the basic exercise, followed by 10 repetitions of the added extension.

- Come back to neutral and take a few deep breaths, resting for 10 seconds. Move into **Chair Pigeon** (page 42) for five deep breaths per leg.

- Return to neutral, and take a few deep breaths, resting for 10 seconds, before moving into **Elbow Rotations** (page 24). Work through the full exercise for five reps. Return to neutral, and rest for 10 seconds, then repeat a second set of five reps. Bring your arms down to neutral.

- Rest for 10 seconds. Move into **Cobra Pose** (page 32), holding here for five deep breaths before releasing into neutral.

- Rest for 10 seconds. Finish out your session with two sets of the **Foot Hover** exercise (page 36) for a total of about one minute.

Day 2

- Begin your workout with **Up and Down Arms** (page 14) for 10 repetitions.

- Bring your arms down, rest for ten seconds, and then move into **Spinal Twist** (page 26) for six repetitions.

- Return to neutral, and take a few deep breaths, resting for 10 seconds. Move into **Core Twists** (page 38), performing the exercise for about 30 seconds. Take a few deep breaths as you rest for 15 seconds, then do one more 30-second set.

- Come back to neutral and take a few deep breaths as you rest for 10 seconds. Move into **Flexing Foot** (page 44), performing 10 repetitions per leg.

- Return to neutral and move into **Eagle Arms** (page 22), going through the exercise once with the right arm over the left and then once more with the left arm over the right.

Day 3

- Begin by moving through **Cactus Pose** (page 12). Hold the pose for five deep breaths, release, then perform one more repetition of the exercise. Return to neutral, and rest for 10 seconds.

- Move into **Head Tilts** (page 18), going through the exercise for three deep breaths per side.

- Come back to neutral and rest for 10 seconds before performing two sets of the **Two Chair Forward Fold** exercise (page 30).

- Come to a standing position behind your chair and take a few deep breaths before moving into **Tree Pose** (page 46), performing the exercise once through on both legs.

- Return to a seated position, take a few deep breaths, and move into **Crunches** (page 40), performing two sets of six repetitions.

Day 4

- Begin with two sets of **Arm Rotations** (page 14), taking a 10-second rest in between sets. Lower your arms to neutral and rest for 10 seconds.

- Perform two sets of the **Shoulder Rolls** exercise (page 20) and come back to neutral. Rest for 10 seconds.

- Move into the **Cat/Cow** exercise (page 28) for five reps. Rest for 10 seconds.

- Perform two sets of the **Foot Hover** exercise (page 36). Return to neutral, and rest for 10 seconds.

- Finish your session with **Quad Lifts** (page 48), performing 10 reps per leg.

Day 5

- Begin with **Elbow Rotations** (page 22), working through the full exercise for five reps. Rest for 10 seconds, then repeat a second set of five reps. Bring your arms down to neutral and rest for 10 seconds.

- Perform two sets of the **Core Twists** exercise (page 38), taking a few deep breaths between sets.

- Move into **Cobra Pose** (page 32). Hold this pose for five deep breaths. Come back to neutral and rest for 10 seconds.

- Stand behind your chair and perform **Tree Pose** (page 46), working the full exercise once through on both legs.

- Return to your chair for five reps of **Sun Breaths** (page 16).

Week 4

Day 1

- Begin your session with five reps of **Sun Breaths** (page 16). Come back to neutral and rest for 10 seconds.

- Move into **Head Tilts** (page 18), moving through the exercise for three deep breaths per side. Rest for 10 seconds.

- Perform two sets of six reps of the **Crunches** exercise (page 40) with a 10-second rest in between sets.

- Stand behind your chair and take a few deep, grounding breaths for about 15 seconds. Perform the **Tree Pose** exercise (page 46) once through on both legs.

- Return to your chair and take a few deep breaths for about 10 seconds. Finish out your session with two sets of the **Core Twists** exercise (page 38), taking a 10-second break in between sets.

Day 2

- Begin with the **Chair Pigeon** stretch (page 42), holding the pose for five deep breaths per leg. Come back to neutral and rest for 10 seconds.

- Move into two full sets of the **Marches** exercise (page 34), taking a 10-second break between sets.

- Return to neutral and take a few deep breaths for about 15 seconds. Move into six reps of **Spinal Twist** (page 26). Rest for 10 seconds.

- Work through the **Elbow Rotations** exercise (page 24) for five reps. Rest for 10 seconds, then repeat a second set of five reps.

- Finish your workout with two sets of **Cactus Pose** (page 12) held for five full breaths per set.

Day 3

- Begin with two sets of **Arm Rotations** (page 14), taking a 10-second rest in between sets.

- Rest for 10 seconds, then work through the **Eagle Arms** exercise (page 22) once with the right arm over the left, then once more with the left arm over the right. Return to neutral and rest for 10 seconds.

- Move into the **Two Chair Forward Fold** (page 30), performing two sets of the full exercise.

- Return to neutral and take a few deep breaths before moving once through the **Flexing Foot** exercise (page 44) with 10 reps per side. Take some deep, grounding breaths for about 15 seconds.

- Close it out with two sets of the **Foot Hover** exercise (page 36), pausing to take a few deep breaths between sets.

Day 4

- Work through two sets of 10 reps per leg of the **Quad Lifts** exercise (page 48), resting for 10 seconds between sets. Rest for 15 seconds.

- Move into two sets of the **Crunches** exercise (page 40), taking a 10-second break between sets.

- Return to neutral and take a few deep breaths, resting for 15 seconds before coming into **Cobra Pose** (page 32). Hold the pose for five deep breaths. Return to neutral and rest for 10 seconds.

- Move into **Head Tilts** (page 18) for three deep breaths per side. Rest for 10 seconds in neutral.

- Finish up with two sets of the full **Up and Down Arms** exercise (page 10).

Day 5

- Begin with two sets of **Cactus Pose** (page 12) held for five deep breaths per set. Rest in neutral for 10 seconds.

- Move into two sets of the **Shoulder Rolls** exercise (page 20).

- Rest for 10 seconds, then move into two sets of the **Cat/Cow** exercise (page 28). Return to neutral and take a few deep breaths, resting for 10 seconds.

- Move to two sets of the full **Marches** exercise (page 34). Rest for 10 seconds.

- Move into **Chair Pigeon** (page 42) to close out your session, holding the pose for five deep breaths per side.

Key Takeaways

The most important thing to remember as you're getting accustomed to these beginner-level yoga exercises is to listen to your body. If something feels wrong, that's a signal for you to stop what you're doing and make a modification. Remember that these exercises are designed to make you feel good, not to cause you any sort of pain or discomfort. There is a difference between feeling a nice stretch and feeling pain in your muscles or on your joints.

Make sure that you're moving through these exercises slowly, especially the first time you go through an exercise. This will help ensure that you're using the proper form and following all the steps.

A lot of people, especially those who are new to yoga, forget to breathe as they're moving through yoga poses. Yoga exercises rely on proper breathwork to ground your body and mind and make sure you execute the positions properly. It may take some time to get used to, but the more focus you place on your breathwork, the more intuitive it will become as you start to move on to more challenging chair yoga exercises.

Chapter 4:

Intermediate Level Challenge

What to Expect

Once you feel comfortable with the beginner-level poses and want to move on to more challenging ones, make sure you're continuing to listen to your body and honor its limits. These poses will feel different from the beginner-level poses, so it's important to modify poses or take breaks as needed. With consistent practice, you'll gradually build strength, flexibility, and endurance to feel comfortable at the intermediate level.

Intermediate-level poses will introduce you to more complexity, requiring increased balance, flexibility, and strength. You'll explore poses that focus on different muscle groups that will help build your capabilities for everyday essential tasks like comfortably moving from a sitting to a standing position.

These poses will also rely more on maintaining proper alignment and posture as they become more intricate, helping you to build the foundation for good posture in your everyday life and avoid injury.

You'll also start to work on smoother transitions between poses, enhancing the flow of your practice. Additionally, the poses will challenge you to hold for longer periods of time to help build your endurance and strength. Some poses may be repeated multiple times or integrated into longer sequences to increase intensity as well.

Flow sequences involve moving from one pose to another in a fluid, continuous manner, improving agility, coordination, and stamina. Flowing with your breathwork also helps you stay present and enhances the mind-body connection.

Intermediate Poses for Arms

Goddess Pose

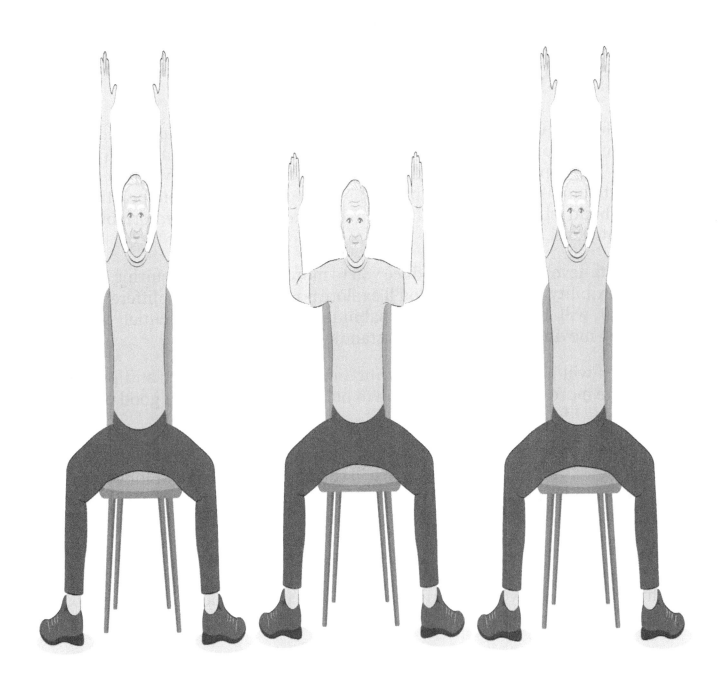

Set up:

- Place your chair in a comfortable area to practice chair yoga, and make sure you have sufficient room to move freely.

Instructions:

- Sit comfortably in your chair with your palms resting on your thighs.

- On an inhale, bring your thighs outward so that your feet are on either side of your chair's legs and pointed outward.

- Bring your hands up on your thighs, toward your hips. Exhale and gently press on your thighs, moving them further outward until you feel a stretch.

- Inhale and bring your arms up over your head so that your fingers are pointed toward the ceiling and your palms are facing each other. Your hands should be in line with your shoulders.

- Exhale and bend at the elbow, bringing your arms down so that they're at a 90-degree angle with your upper arms at shoulder height.

- Have your palms facing forward. Hold here for five full, deep breaths.

- Inhale and raise your arms up again and hold for another five breaths.

- To release the pose, on an exhale, bring your palms down to rest on your thighs and your legs together. Stay in this position for five deep breaths.

- Repeat this sequence twice more.

Key considerations:

- To ensure that your feet are grounded on the floor throughout this exercise, you may need to scoot forward on your chair.

- Your feet should always be in line with your knees; a good way to check is by making sure your ankles are directly under your knees, and your toes are pointed in the same direction as your knees and thighs.

- When raising your arms above your head, check that your shoulders are relaxed by letting them drop down and back.

Front Facing Arm Raises

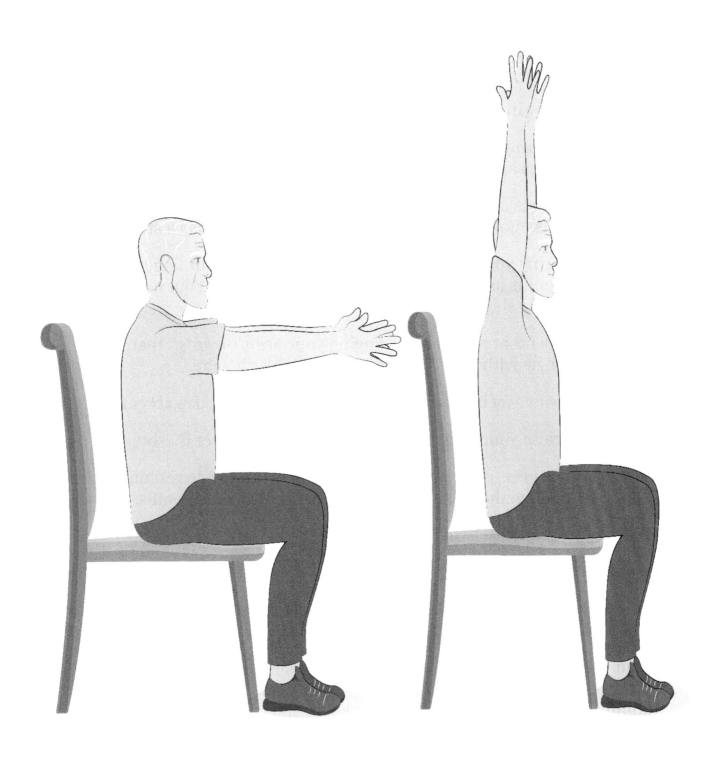

Set up:

- Bring your chair to your designated chair yoga spot, and check that there is nothing that will get in the way of your movement.

Instructions:

- Sit comfortably in your chair with your palms resting on your thighs.

- Scoot forward slightly to create some gap between the backrest of the chair and your back.

- Raise your arms straight out in front of you with your fingers pointed outward and your palms facing each other.

- Hold here for a breath.

- Inhale and raise your arms up over your head, maintaining the same hand alignment.

- Exhale and lower your arms back down to their previous position so that they are straight in front of you.

- Repeat this sequence 10 times, lifting your arms up as you inhale and bringing them down to shoulder height as you exhale.

- Make sure to keep a fluid motion and let your breath guide your speed.

- To release the pose, lower your palms down to your thighs on an exhale.

Key considerations:

- Throughout the exercise, maintain a slight bend at the elbow to avoid locking the joints.

- If you want to increase the difficulty of this exercise, you can hold light weights (about two or three pounds). If you don't have weights, you can use cans of beans.

- Periodically check in to see that you're not carrying tension in your shoulders and neck by dropping your shoulders down and back.

Palm Tree Side Bend

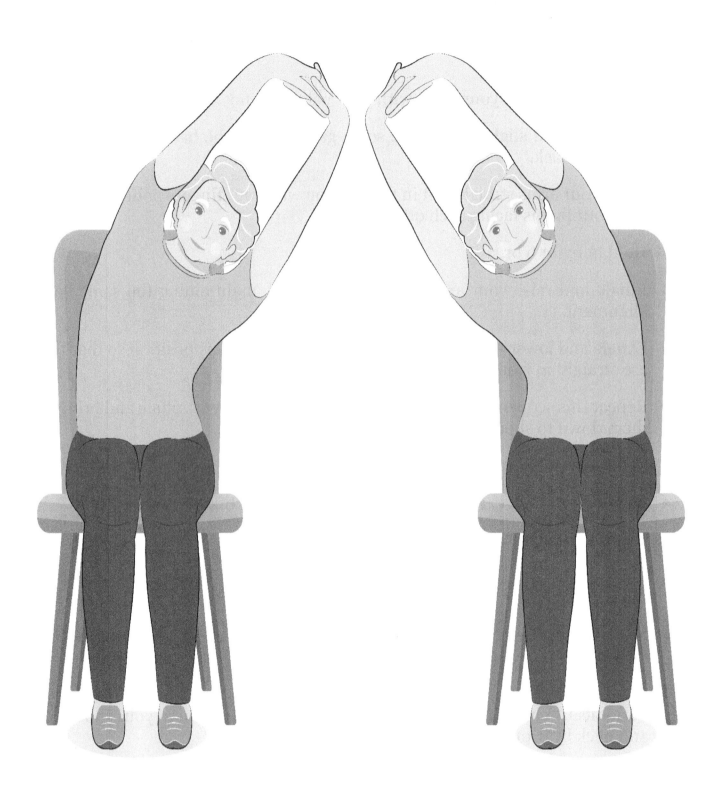

Set up:

- Bring your chair to a comfortable, open area to practice chair yoga.

Instructions:

- Sit comfortably in your chair and take a few deep breaths.

- On an inhale, raise your arms over your head and interlace your fingers with your palms facing upward or as close to upward as you can get. Exhale.

- Inhale and slowly bend your torso to the left, lengthening the stretch in your arms as you reach your interlaced hands to your left.

- Exhale and slowly return to the center with your arms reaching straight above you.

- Inhale and slowly bend to your right, reaching with your arms and feeling the stretch in your left arm.

- Exhale and come back to the center.

- Repeat this sequence 10 times, bending to one side as you inhale and coming back to the center as you exhale, alternating between the two sides.

- Make sure to keep a fluid motion and let your breath guide your speed.

- To release the pose, unclasp your fingers and circle your arms back down on an exhale. Rest your palms on your thighs.

Key considerations:

- Make sure your head, neck, spine, and arms are in alignment throughout this exercise.

- When raising your arms above your head, check that your shoulders are relaxed by letting them drop down and back.

- Make sure you're actively engaging your core throughout this exercise to prevent putting strain on your back.

Knee Claps

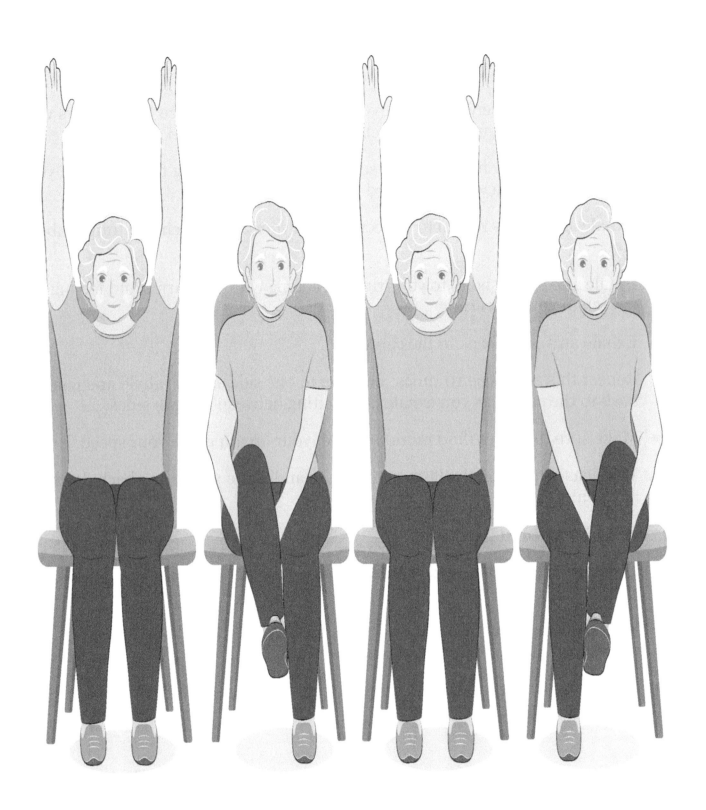

Set up:

- Bring your chair to a comfortable and open area to practice chair yoga. Make sure you have sufficient space to move your arms around freely.

Instructions:

- Sit comfortably in your chair with your arms by your sides.

- On an inhale, extend your arms out to the sides and then up over your head with your fingers pointing toward the ceiling and palms facing each other.

- Exhale and bring your arms down as you lift your right leg up, maintaining the bend at the knee, and clap your hands under your lifted knee.

- Inhale and bring your arms back up over your head and lower your foot back to the floor.

- Exhale and repeat the clapping motion with your left leg by bringing your arms down as you lift your left leg up to clap under the left leg.

- Repeat this sequence, alternating legs, for about thirty seconds before slowing to a stop.

- To release, bring your feet to the floor and place your hands on your thighs.

- Repeat this exercise once through.

Key considerations:

- Make sure to engage your core throughout this exercise and maintain a straight back. When you clap your hands under your knees, you can bend a bit at the hips instead of hunching the back.

- Your breath and movements should be fluid; allow your breathing to guide your movements. As you inhale, lift your arms up, and as you exhale, clap your hands under your lifted knee.

Intermediate Poses for the Neck and Shoulders

Fish Pose

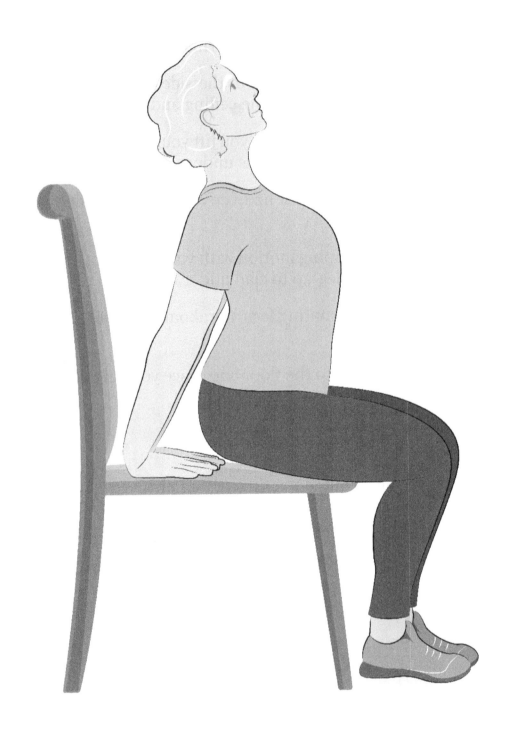

Set up:

- Bring your chair to a comfortable and open area to practice chair yoga, making sure that you can engage in a full range of motion without bumping into anything.

Instructions:

- Sit comfortably toward the edge of your chair and take a few deep breaths.

- On an exhale, slowly lean back into the chair to place your hands close to where the backrest and the seat of the chair meet.

- Your torso should be in a diagonal position, as opposed to upright.

- Inhale deeply, and when you exhale, expand your chest, as if you have a rope attached to your ribcage that is pulling you toward the ceiling.

- Bring your gaze up to the ceiling as you feel your chest opening up even more.

- Let your shoulders roll back and drop fully to increase the stretch.

- Hold this pose for six full, deep breaths.

- To release, slowly bring your torso back to upright position, bringing your gaze forward. Bring your palms back on to your thighs.

- Repeat this exercise once through.

Key considerations:

- When arching your upper back, instead of dropping your head back, think about lengthening the neck and sending your gaze upward.

- During this pose, it can be tempting to force the arch in your back; instead of doing so, focus on expanding your chest and relaxing your neck and shoulders. This will allow you to feel a nice stretch in your chest area and help release any tension you may be carrying in your upper body.

- Grab a pillow, rolled-up towel, or blanket, and place it at the back of the seat to have additional support if needed.

Revolved Chair Pose

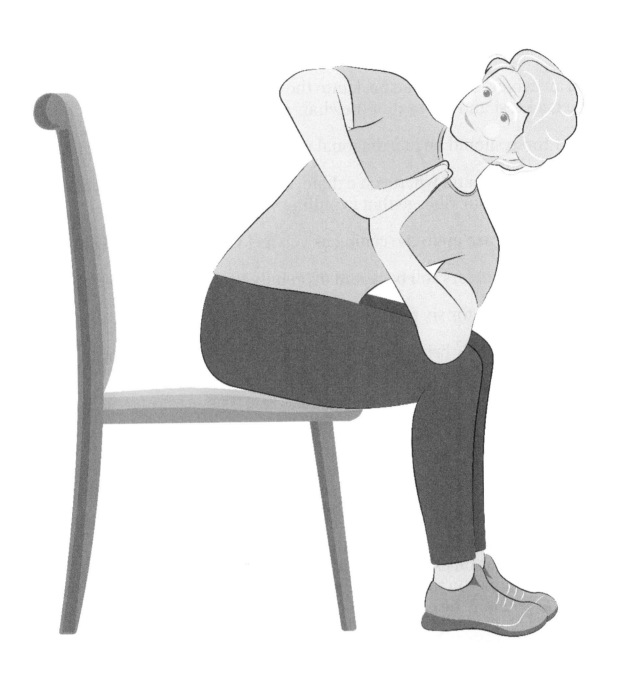

Set up:

- Bring your chair to your designated chair yoga area and make sure there are no objects around that will get in the way of your movement.

Instructions:

- Sit comfortably in your chair with your hands in your lap.

- On an inhale, bring your palms together in front of your chest with your fingers pointed upward to form a prayer pose.

- Exhale and twist your upper body to the right as you keep your palms together.

- Bring your left elbow to your right thigh, just above the knee. You can hook your elbow on the outer side of your thigh for support.

- Inhale and reach your right elbow back as far as is comfortable.

- Exhale and slowly twist your neck further to the right, bringing your gaze upwards as far as is comfortable.

- Hold this pose for ten more deep breaths.

- To release, on an inhale, gently release from the twist, starting with the head, and slowly bring your torso back to an upright seated position. Follow this with placing your hands back in your lap.

- Take five deep breaths to relax and ten repeat once more on the other side.

Key considerations:

- Make sure to maintain a tall spine and neck throughout the exercise. Engage your core to help keep your posture aligned.

- Make sure to move into and out of the twists slowly.

- Breathing deeply into each twist will help control the pace of your movements.

- Resist forcing the twist; instead, twist as far as feels comfortable.

Gate Pose

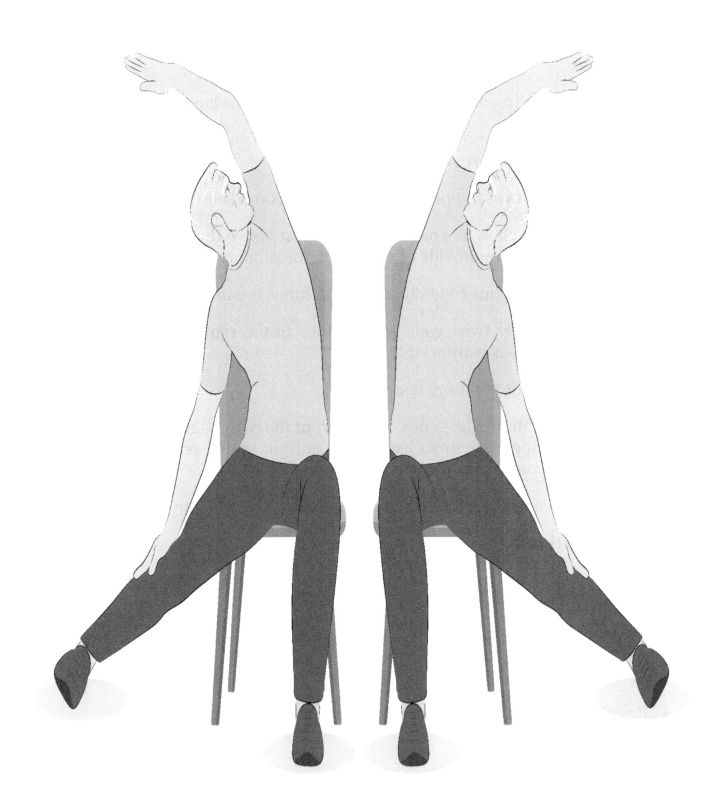

Set up:

- Bring your chair to your designated chair yoga space and make sure you have enough room to move freely.

Instructions:

- Sit comfortably in the right corner of your chair.

- Place your weight on your left sit bones.

- On an inhale, stretch your right leg to your right side so that the inner side of the sole of your right foot is on the floor and pointed forward.

- Exhale and lengthen through the hips and legs further.

- Inhale and bring your right palm to the outer side of your right shin, bending your torso to your right side as well. Exhale.

- Inhale and reach your left arm over your head and to the right.

- Exhale and extend the arm further as you bring your gaze up toward the ceiling.

- Hold this position for six deep breaths as you feel a nice stretch in your upper body.

- Slowly release the position of your upper body, moving it back to an upright position on an inhale.

- Exhale and bring your right leg up to meet your left leg, and move to the other corner of your chair.

- Repeat this sequence once more on your left side.

Key considerations:

- Think about lengthening the body during this exercise. Your back, arms, and legs should be in elongated positions as opposed to compressed.

- Only move to a position that you feel comfortable in. This pose is meant to stretch your upper body; if you're feeling pressure in your lower back, gently release your position until the feeling subsides.

Elbow-to-Knee

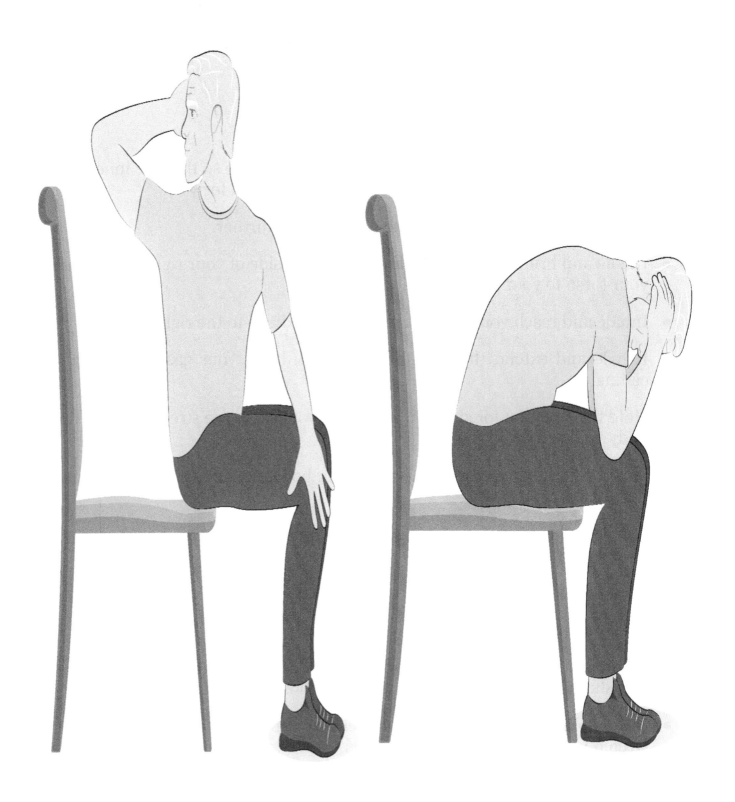

Set up:

- Bring your chair to your designated chair yoga area, making sure that you have sufficient room to move.

Instructions:

- Sit comfortably in your chair with your palms resting on your thighs.

- Place your left hand on the outer side of your right knee and straighten out your left arm as you press your left hand into your right knee.

- Feel free to grab your right knee if that's easier.

- On an inhale, bring your right hand to the back of your head with your elbow pointing out to the side.

- Gently twist to the right as you stretch your elbow back.

- Turn your head, letting your gaze follow your elbow.

- Exhale and slowly bring your raised elbow down to your right knee as you release your left hand.

- Let your head drop by relaxing your neck.

- Inhale deeply, and on the exhale, gently press slightly forward and down at the base of your neck, increasing the stretch in your neck without forcing the chin into the chest.

- Inhale and slowly come back up to a neutral seated position by lowering your palms to your thighs and then repeat this sequence four times.

- Come back to the starting position and then repeat the sequence five times on the left side.

Key considerations:

- Engage your core throughout this exercise, and check that you aren't carrying any tension in your shoulders or neck by letting your shoulders drop down and back.

- Resist forcing the twist; instead, twist as far as feels comfortable.

Intermediate Poses for Chest and Back

Forward Fold

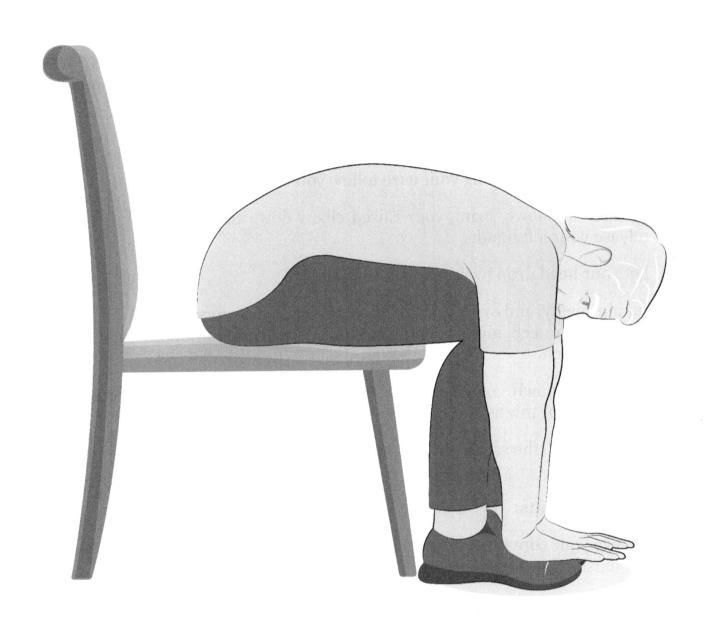

Set up:

- Bring your chair to your designated chair yoga space, and make sure that there is nothing that will get in the way of your movement.

- If you would like more chest support during this pose, you can also use a pillow, rolled-up blanket, or towel.

Instructions:

- Sit comfortably in your chair.

- If you're using a pillow, place it on your upper thigh area.

- On an inhale, slowly hinge at the hips, bringing your torso forward over your thighs.

- Allow your arms to drop down on the outsides of your legs.

- Drop your torso as far down as is comfortable for you, letting your hands rest on your feet, and your head drop by completely relaxing your neck.

- Feel your spine decompress and the gentle stretch in your back muscles.

- Hold this position for four deep breaths.

- On an inhale, slowly raise your torso back up, engaging your abdominal muscles.

- Feel each vertebra stack atop each other as you roll up to a sitting position and come out of the pose.

- Rest your palms on your thighs and then repeat this exercise once through.

Key considerations:

- Once you are in the forward fold position, you can bring your attention to your body, focusing on one body part at a time to make sure that you are not carrying any tension.

- Your body should be completely relaxed while in the forward fold pose; allow your arms, shoulders, head, and neck to relax into a dropped position.

Downward Dog

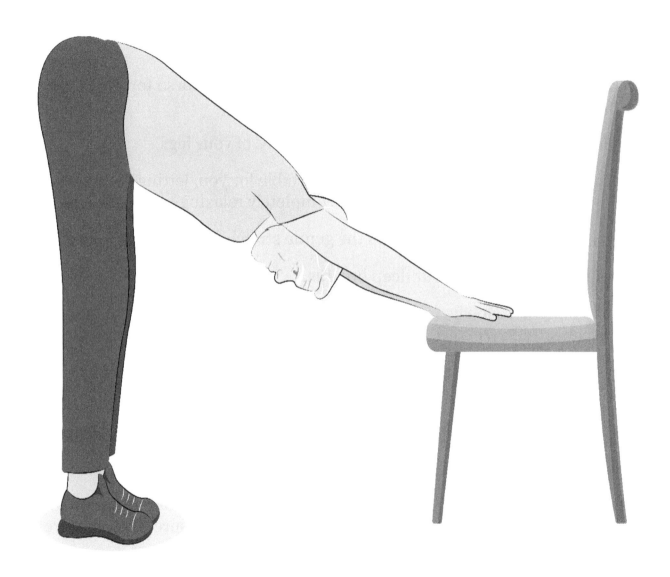

Set up:

- Place your chair against a wall, and make sure that you have enough room in front of the wall to move freely.

- During this pose, it's best to either be barefoot or wear athletic shoes with a good grip to avoid potential slipping.

Instructions:

- Stand facing your chair and take a few deep breaths.

- On an exhale, lower your palms to the seat of the chair, bending at the hips and keeping your back straight.

- Slowly walk your feet back until your spine feels elongated and your arms are on either side of your ears, fully extended.

- Maintain a slight bend in your knees and press your heels into the floor to lift your hips slightly as you feel a stretch in your hamstrings.

- Hold this pose for six deep breaths, feeling your torso lengthen and the vertebra in your spine decompress.

- To release, slowly walk your feet forward until you return to a standing position.

- Repeat this exercise once through.

Key considerations:

- Engage your core during this exercise to help keep your spine straight. Make sure that your head is in line with your back and arms while you're in the downward dog position.

- Maintain a slight bend at the knees to avoid locking or overextending them. While this pose primarily decompresses your spine, you will also likely feel a light stretch in your hamstrings.

Wide-Leg Forward Fold

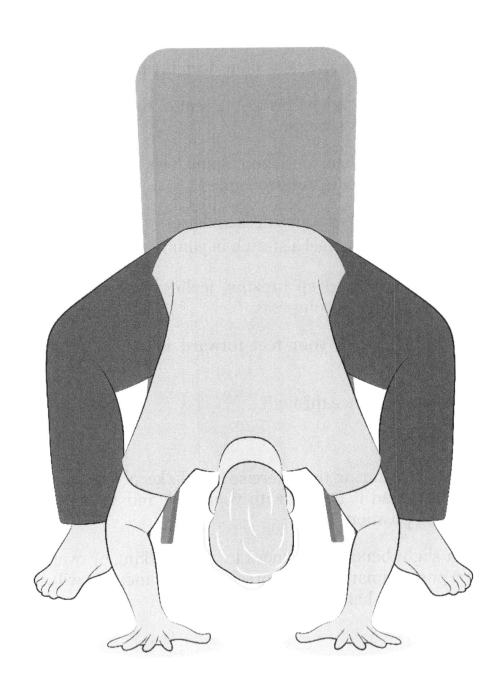

Set up:

- Bring your chair to a comfortable area for chair yoga, making sure you have sufficient space to move.

Instructions:

- Sit comfortably in your chair.

- Widen your stance so that your thighs, knees, and feet are opened and pointed outward.

- Make sure you're still maintaining a 90-degree angle with your legs.

- Inhale and lift your torso upwards, thinking about lengthening your spine.

- Exhale and bring your torso forward and down between your thighs, bending at the hips and maintaining a straight back.

- Let your hands drop to the floor, and your head hang down.

- Feel your spine expand and lower bank lengthen.

- Hold this position for five deep breaths.

- Engage your core, and slowly lift your torso back up to a sitting position to release.

- Repeat this exercise once through.

Key considerations:

- You may want to sit more toward the edge of your chair if it's more comfortable for you to move into a wider seated stance.

- Make sure to move through this exercise slowly and remember to breathe throughout to prevent any potential lightheadedness.

- You may find it easier to place a yoga block in front of you to place your hands on instead of the floor and gradually improve your range of motion.

Tabletop Torso Circles

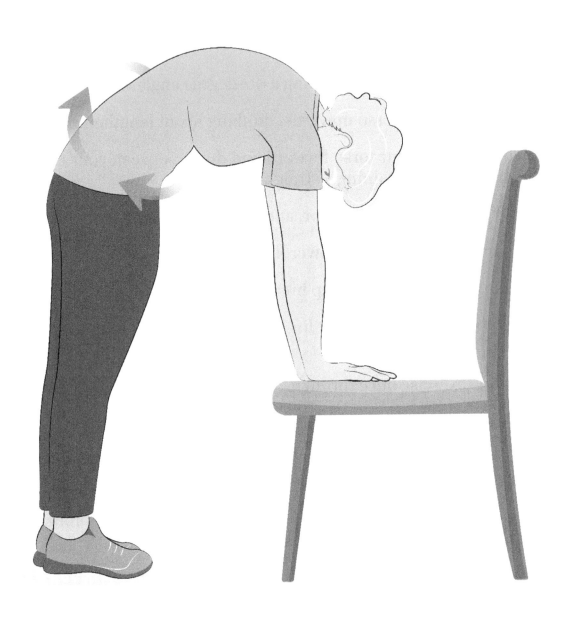

Set up:

- Bring your chair to a quiet, open area to practice chair yoga, and make sure you have room to stand and move in front of your chair.

Instructions:

- Stand facing the seat of your chair, a couple of feet away from it.

- Bending at the hips, slowly bring your torso down 90 degrees and extend your arms down so that your palms are resting on the seat of your chair.

- On an inhale, engage your core and begin to rotate your torso by lifting it up, then left, then down, and then right, in a circular motion.

- Continue to slowly circle your torso for ten deep breaths.

- Slow to a stop, then begin moving in the opposite direction, remembering to let your breathing guide you.

- Move in this direction for another ten deep breaths.

- To release, slowly raise your torso to a standing position.

- Repeat this exercise once through.

Key considerations:

- Your breath and movements should be fluid; allow your breathing to guide your movements.

- Make sure that your head is in line with your back and your shoulders are directly above your hands.

- Maintain a slight bend at the knees to avoid locking or overextending them. While this pose primarily decompresses your spine, you will also likely feel a light stretch in your hamstrings.

Intermediate Poses for Abs

Boat Pose

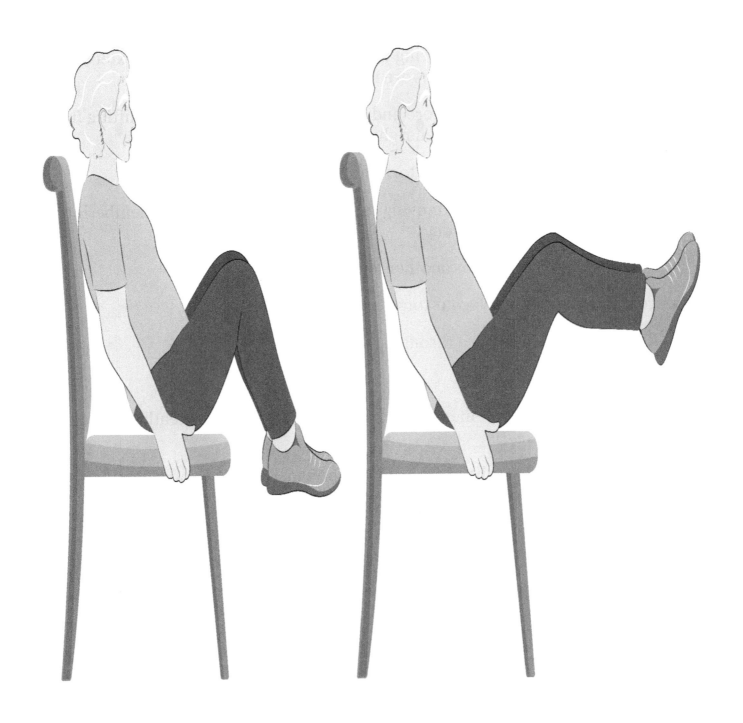

Set up:

- Bring your chair to a comfortable, open area to practice chair yoga, making sure you have sufficient room to move.

Instructions:

- Sit comfortably in your chair, about halfway down the middle of the seat.

- Grab the sides of the seat of the chair firmly with your hands.

- Engage your core and slowly bend at the hips to lean backward, bringing your torso back while maintaining a straight spine.

- Lift your feet off the floor until they are at the seat's height level or as high as possible, keeping your knees bent and pointing your toes.

- Hold here for four deep breaths.

- Take a deep breath in and extend your legs forward, maintaining a bend at the knees so that your legs are at about a 140-degree angle.

- Hold here for four deep breaths.

- To release, on an exhale, lower your feet to the floor and slowly bring your torso upright.

- Repeat this exercise once through.

Key considerations:

- To help with balance, you can grab the sides of your chair as you're lifting your feet off the floor.

- Your upper back can touch the back of your chair but avoid leaning your weight into the back of the chair too much. Your core should be keeping your upper body in its proper position.

Hover Leg Tilts

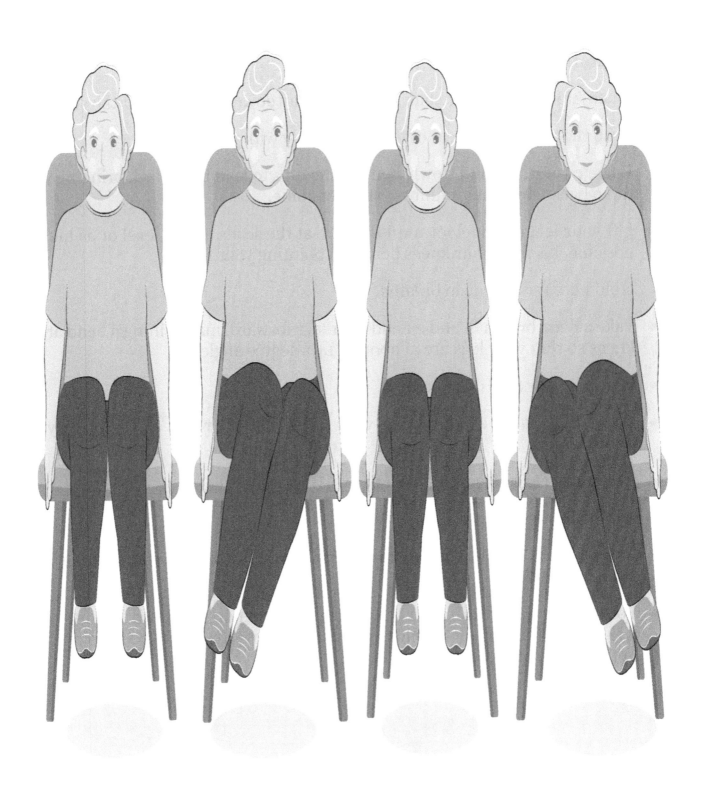

Set up:

- Bring your chair to your designated chair yoga area, making sure you have enough room around you to comfortably move.

Instructions:

- Sit comfortably in your chair with your shoulders relaxed.

- Keeping your back straight, on inhale, lift your feet off the floor a few inches by engaging your core muscles.

- Make sure that your legs are together so that they are connected all the way down to your feet.

- Exhale and slowly tilt your legs to the right as far as is comfortable for you while keeping your upper body stationary.

- Inhale and bring your feet back to the center, still a few inches off the floor.

- Exhale and tilt your legs to the left as far as is comfortable for you while keeping your upper body stationary.

- Inhale and bring your feet back to the center, still a few inches off the floor.

- Repeat this sequence for ten repetitions.

- To release, bring your feet to the center and lower them to the floor.

Key considerations:

- Make sure to engage your core throughout this exercise so that you aren't putting any strain on your lower back. You should feel this exercise on the sides of your core and also on your thighs.

- To help with balance, you can grab the sides of your chair as you're lifting your feet off the floor.

- With many abdominal exercises, people tend to restrict their breathing. This is especially true when you are in a position that works your abs. To make sure that you're breathing properly, bring your attention to your rib cage. As you inhale, you should be able to feel and see your rib cage expanding. As you exhale, you should feel and see it contract.

Bicycles

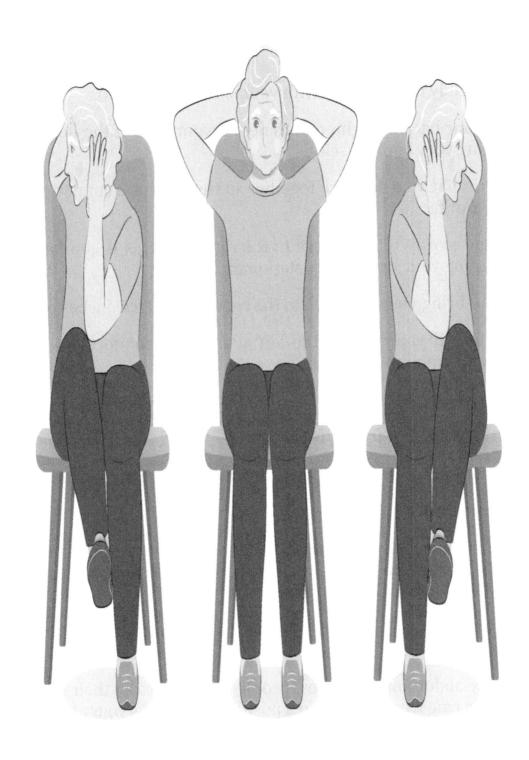

Set up:

- Place your chair in a comfortable area to practice chair yoga, making sure that there are no objects that will get in the way of your movement.

Instructions:

- Sit comfortably in your chair and bring your hands behind your head, interlacing your fingers.

- Engage your core and bring your right elbow down while bringing your left knee up to meet each other.

- Gently tap the elbow and the knee together or bring them as close as you can get them together.

- Then slowly release your leg back down and bring your torso back up to the starting position while keeping your fingers interlaced behind your head.

- Repeat this on the same side for five repetitions.

- On the last repetition, hold in the position where your elbow and knee meet for five seconds before releasing.

- To release, bring your feet to the floor, bring your torso upright, and lower your palms to your thighs.

- Repeat this sequence once more on the other side by bringing your left elbow to meet your right knee.

Key considerations:

- Remember to breathe throughout this exercise; it can be easy to forget to practice proper breathing during a workout, especially while working your abs.

- When you're moving to touch your knee with your elbow, instead of forcing your head down, allow your head to come down however far is comfortable for you while supporting an extended neck with your interlaced fingers.

- Also, check to see if you are carrying tension in your shoulders. If you feel that you are, drop them down and back so that they are relaxed.

Plank Pose

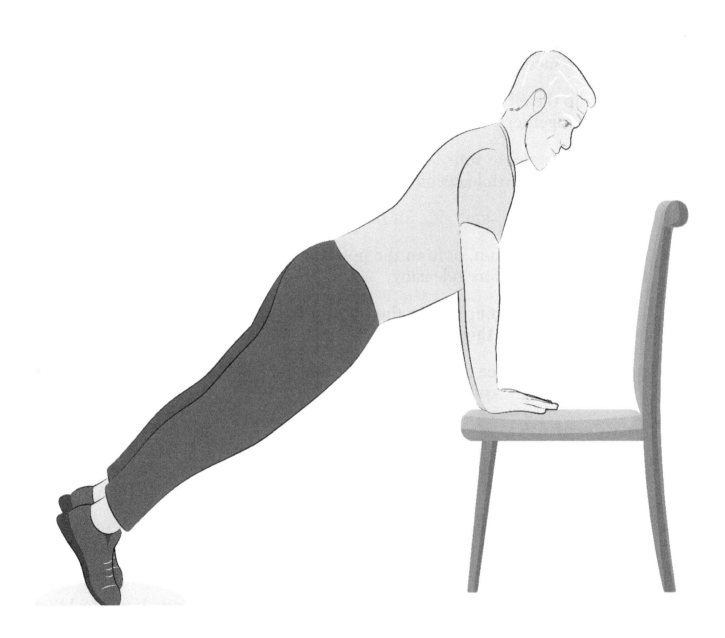

Set up:

- Bring your chair to your designated chair yoga area and make sure you have sufficient room in front of your chair.

Instructions:

- Stand a couple of feet away from your chair, facing the seat.

- On an exhale, hinge at the hips to lower your upper body closer to the chair and place the palms of your hands on the seat of the chair.

- Make sure your arms are straight, with your shoulders directly above your hands.

- Inhale, engage your core and walk your feet back until you are in a plank position with your arms supporting your weight and perpendicular to the seat of the chair.

- The weight of your lower body should be supported by the balls of your feet.

- Make sure that you keep your core muscles engaged to keep a straight back, and keep your head in line with your spine to avoid straining your neck.

- Hold this position for five full, deep breaths.

- To release, walk your feet toward the chair and come back up to a standing position.

Key considerations:

- You can place the back of your chair against a wall to ensure the chair won't slip when you lean your weight on it.

- If you are finding it hard to complete the plank pose, try placing yoga blocks or pillows under your knees to rest your knees on these and gradually build up your strength to complete the pose without any support.

Intermediate Poses for Legs

Triangle Pose

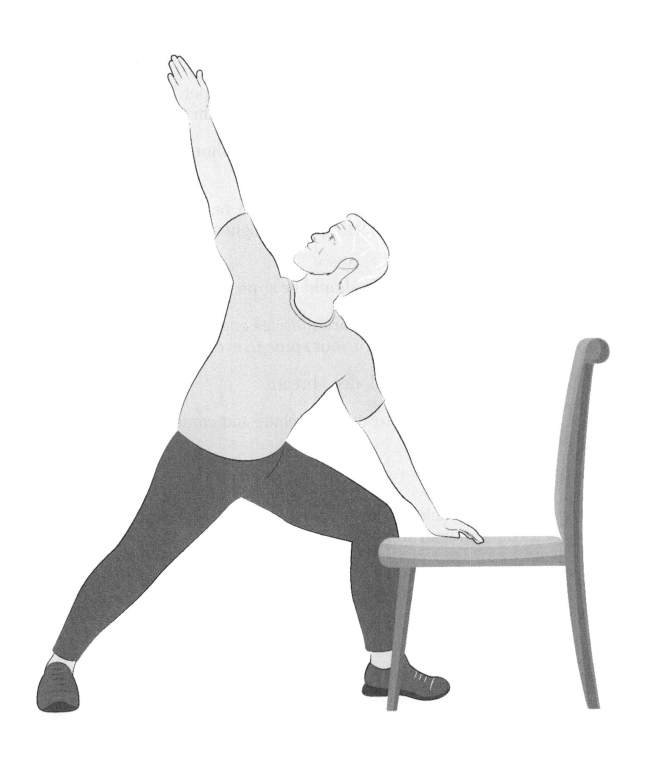

Set up:

- Bring your chair to your designated chair yoga area, making sure that you have sufficient room to stand and move in front of your chair.

Instructions:

- Stand in front of your chair facing the seat.

- Place your left foot directly in front of the chair and bring your right foot back and angled out.

- Keep a nice bend in your left leg while making sure your right leg is fully extended.

- Your left foot should point toward the chair whereas the right foot should be perpendicular to the chair.

- On an exhale, drop down slightly until you have a slight bend in your left knee while keeping the right leg fully extended out to reach your left hand down to rest on the seat of the chair.

- Inhale and reach your right arm up toward the ceiling, letting your gaze follow your fingertips.

- Hold this pose for ten deep breaths.

- To release, slowly come back to standing.

- Repeat once more on the other side by placing your right foot in front of the chair, bringing your left foot back, right hand down to rest on the seat of the chair, and left arm up toward the ceiling, letting your gaze follow your fingertips.

Key considerations:

- You can place your chair against a wall to help prevent any potential slipping of the chair while leaning your weight on it.

- When bending at the knee, your knee should be directly above your ankle.

Side Leg Lifts

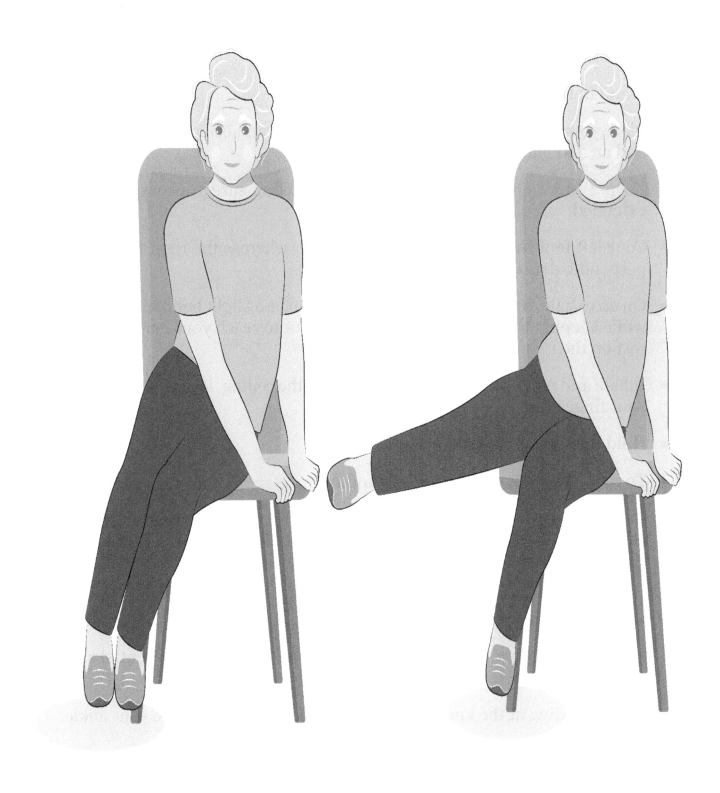

Set up:

- Bring your chair to a comfortable and open area for chair yoga, and check that you have enough room to extend your legs in all directions while seated.

Instructions:

- Sit comfortably on the right edge of your chair, facing forward.

- Grab onto the left edge of the chair's seat and bring your feet together to the right of the chair.

- Reach your right leg out to the right side so that your leg is extended and the left edge of the sole of your right foot is resting on the floor with your toes still pointed forward.

- On an inhale, moving from the hip, lift your right leg so that your foot is about a foot off the floor.

- On an exhale, lower your foot back to the floor.

- Continue raising and lowering your leg for ten repetitions.

- To release, sit in the middle of your chair and bring your legs together in front of you. Rest your hands on your thighs.

- After a few deep breaths, move to the left side of your chair and repeat the sequence once more with your left leg.

Key considerations:

- Engage your entire active leg during the lifts. You should feel the exercise in your thighs, hips, and glutes.

- Only lift your leg up as far as comfortably possible while keeping a straight back. Avoid tilting to one side to lift your leg up higher.

Warrior II

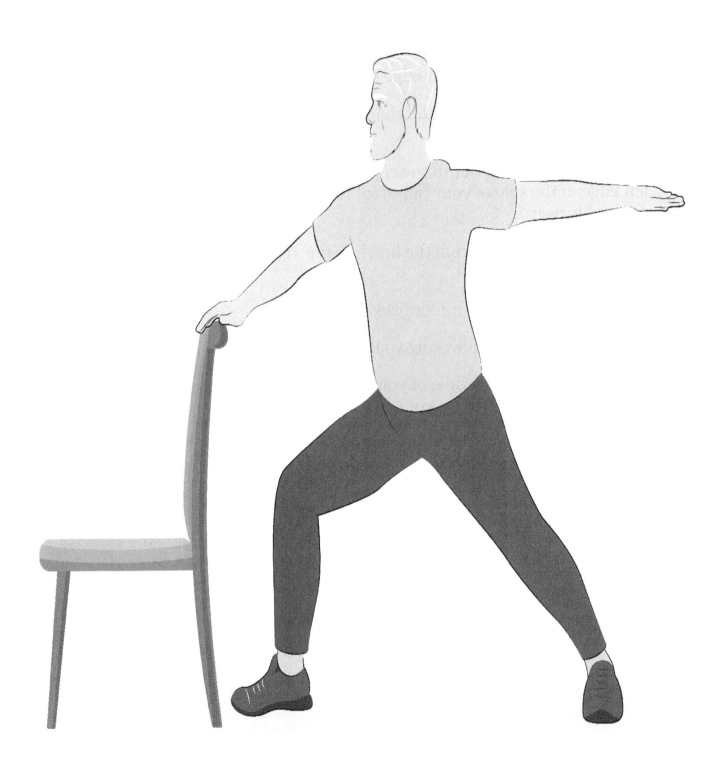

Set up:

- Bring your chair to a comfortable and open area to practice chair yoga. Make sure that you have enough room to move with a wide stance behind your chair.

Instructions:

- Stand behind your chair and grab onto the back of the chair with your right hand for support.

- Bring your left leg back and open your stance so that your left foot is positioned perpendicularly to the chair and your right foot is facing the same direction the chair is facing.

- Drop down slightly until you have a slight bend in your right knee while keeping the left leg fully extended out.

- Keeping your gaze forward, lift your left arm out to shoulder level and stretch it toward the back until you feel your chest opening up.

- Hold here for five deep breaths.

- Bring your back foot forward to meet your forward foot and bring your arms to your sides as you come out of the position.

- Repeat once more on the other side.

Key considerations:

- When bending at the knee, your knee should be directly above your ankle.

- You can place the front of your chair against a wall to ensure the chair won't slip when you lean your weight on it.

- As you become more confident with this pose, try repeating it without holding the chair.

Sit-to-Stand

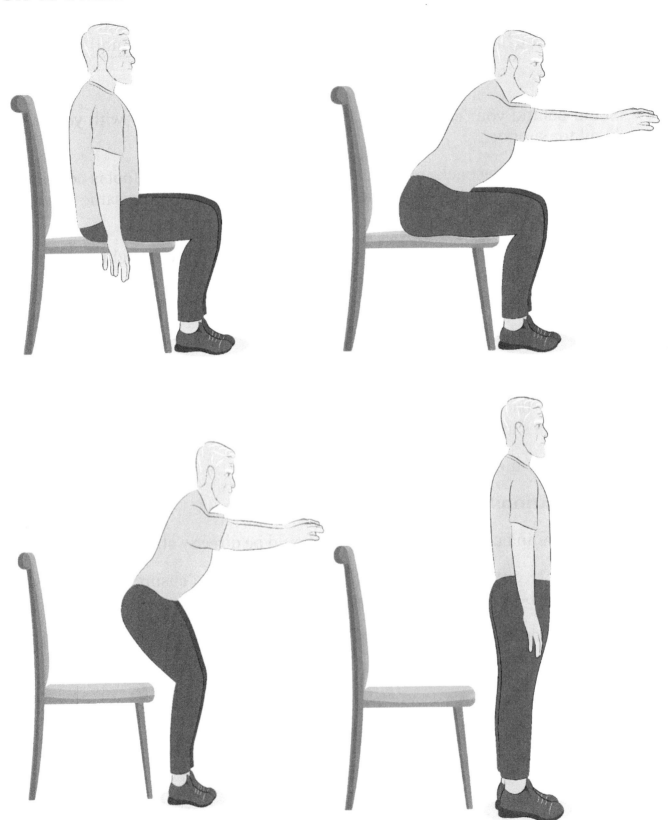

Set up:

- Bring your chair to an open and comfortable area to practice chair yoga, making sure that you have sufficient room to stand in front of your chair.

Instructions:

- Sit comfortably in your chair with your palms resting on your thighs.

- Take a few deep breaths.

- Bring your torso slightly forward and shift your weight to your feet.

- Feel the connection of your feet with the floor as you press them onto the floor.

- Engage your leg muscles and extend your arms straight out in front of you with your palms facing the floor.

- Slowly raise your body from the chair until you are in a standing position.

- From here, slowly bend at the knees and hips, maintaining a straight spine as you hinge your torso slightly forward until you return to a seated position in your chair.

- Repeat this exercise six times, remembering to breathe and move slowly through the movements.

- To release, remain in your ending seated position.

Key considerations:

- You can place your chair against a wall if you're worried about it slipping at all.

- Go slow with this exercise instead of relying heavily on momentum to get the most out of the workout. This exercise helps improve your balance as well as strenghten your leg muscles and joint mobility.

Weekly Routine

Week 1

Day 1
- Begin with the **Goddess Pose** (page 58) for two sets.

- From your neutral-ending position, move into the **Elbow-to-Knee** exercise (page 72) for four reps per side.

- Flow directly into **Bicycles** (page 86), performing five reps per side.

Day 2
- Begin with the **Sit-to-Stand** exercise (page 96), performing two sets of six reps with a 10-second rest between sets.

- From your finishing standing position, move behind your chair and flow into **Warrior II** (page 94) for five deep breaths per side.

- Come back to a seated position and move directly into **Gate Pose** (page 70) for six deep breaths per side.

Day 3
- Begin with the **Forward Fold** (page 74), holding the pose for 10 deep breaths. As you release, stand up and move your second chair out of the way.

- Move into **Triangle Pose** (page 90) for 10 deep breaths per side.

- Release into standing and rest for 15 seconds. From here, move into **Downward Dog** (page 76) for six deep breaths.

Week 2

Day 1
- Begin with **Palm Tree Side Bend** (page 62), performing 10 reps.

- Bring your arms down and flow directly into **Tabletop Torso Circles** (page 80) for 10 repetitions on each side.

- Come down to a neutral seated position and rest for 15 seconds. Move into **Knee Claps** (page 64), working through the exercise for 30 seconds.

- Flow into **Wide-Leg Forward Fold** (page 78), holding the pose for five deep breaths. Come up, then repeat one more set for another five-breath count.

Day 2

- Begin with 10 reps of **Front Facing Arm Raises** (page 60).

- Bring your palms together and flow directly into **Revolved Chair Pose** (page 68), holding the pose for 10 breaths per side.

- Rest for 15 seconds. Move into 10 reps of **Side Leg Lifts** (page 92) per leg.

- From here, flow directly into 2 sets of 10 reps of **Hover Leg Tilts** (page 84), taking a 10-second rest between sets.

Day 3

- Start with **Fish Pose** (page 66), holding for six deep breaths.

- Flow into two sets of four deep breaths held in **Boat Pose** (page 82) with a 10-second rest between sets.

- Come to standing in front of your chair and take a few deep breaths as you take a 15-second break. Move into **Plank Pose** (page 88).

- From here, flow directly into **Downward Dog** (page 76), holding the pose for six deep breaths.

Day 4

- Start with **Warrior II** (page 94), holding for five deep breaths per side.

- Come around to the front of your chair and move into **Triangle Pose** (page 90) for 10 deep breaths per side.

- Flow into the **Plank Pose** (page 88), holding here for five deep breaths.

- Sit down and rest for 15 seconds. Move into **Gate Pose** (page 70), holding for six deep breaths per side.

Week 3

Day 1

- Begin with 10 reps of **Tabletop Torso Circles** (page 80) in one direction and then 10 reps in the opposite direction. Lower back down to a seated position and rest for 10 seconds.

- Move into **Bicycles** (page 86), performing five reps per side.

- Flow directly into **Revolved Chair Pose** (page 68), holding for 10 deep breaths per side.

- Raise your arms into **Palm Tree Side Bends** (page 62), performing 10 reps.

- Bring your arms down and flow into **Side Leg Lifts** (page 92), performing 10 reps per side.

Day 2

- Begin with **Wide-Leg Forward Fold** (page 78), holding for five deep breaths. Come up, then perform one more rep for another five-breath count.

- As you come up, flow directly into **Boat Pose** (page 82), performing two sets of a four-breath count with a 10-second rest between sets.

- Flow into **Fish Pose** (page 66), holding the pose for six breaths.

- Return to neutral and take a 10-second rest. Move into **Elbow-to-Knee** (page 72) for four reps per side.

- Flow into **Goddess Pose** (page 58) for two sets.

Day 3

- Begin with **Forward Fold** (page 74), holding here for 10 deep breaths.

- Moving the second chair away, come to stand behind your chair and move into **Warrior II** (page 94) for five breaths per side.

- Sit in your chair and rest for 10 seconds. Move into **Knee Claps** (page 64) for 30 seconds.

- Flow directly into **Sit to Stand** (page 96), performing two sets of six reps with a 10-second rest between sets.

- Finish out by sitting back down and flowing into **Front Facing Arm Raises** (page 60) for 10 reps.

Day 4

- Begin with **Hover Leg Tilts** (page 84), performing two sets of 10 reps with a 10-second rest between sets.

- From here, flow into **Side Leg Lifts** (page 92), performing 10 reps per side.

- Take a 10-second break before moving into **Fish Pose** (page 66) for six deep breaths.

- Flow directly into **Gate Pose** (page 70), holding for six deep breaths per side.

- Come back to neutral and rest for 10 seconds. Finish out with 10 reps of **Palm Tree Side Bends** (page 62).

Week 4

Day 1

- Start with **Plank Pose** (page 88), holding for five deep breaths.

- From here, flow directly into **Triangle Pose** (page 90) for 10 deep breaths per side.

- Sit down, taking a 10-second break. Move into **Bicycles** (page 86) for five reps per side.

- Take a 10-second break, and move into **Tabletop Torso Circles** (page 80), performing 10 repetitions in each direction.

- Come to a stop and flow into **Revolved Chair Pose** (page 68) for 10 breaths per side.

Day 2

- Start with **Front Facing Arm Raises** (page 60) for ten reps.

- Bring your arms down and flow into **Knee Claps** (page 64) for 30 seconds.

- From here, flow into **Wide-Leg Forward Fold** (page 78), holding for five breaths. Come up, then repeat one more rep for another five-breath count.

- As you come up, flow into **Fish Pose** (page 66), holding here for six breaths.

- Grab your second chair and finish out with **Forward Fold** (page 74), holding for 10 deep breaths.

Day 3

- Begin with **Hover Leg Tilts** (page 84), performing two sets of 10 reps with a 10-second rest between sets.

- Stand and move directly into **Triangle Pose** (page 90) for 10 breaths per side.

- From here, flow directly into **Plank Pose** (page 88), holding for five deep breaths.

- Flow directly into **Downward Dog** (page 76), holding for six breaths.

- Sit back down and finish out your session with **Gate Pose** (page 70), holding for six breaths per side.

Day 4

- Begin with **Goddess Pose** (page 58), moving through the exercise for two sets.

- Bring your arms down and flow into **Boat Pose** (page 82), holding here for four deep breaths. Take a 10-second break, then repeat the sequence for a second set.

- Release to neutral and move directly into **Sit to Stand** (page 96), performing two sets of six reps with a 10-second rest between sets.

- From standing, flow into **Downward Dog** (page 76), holding the pose for six deep breaths.

- Sit back down, take a 10-second rest, and then move into the **Elbow-to-Knee** exercise (page 72) for four reps per side.

Key Takeaways

Intermediate chair yoga offers a deeper exploration of poses and sequences, building upon the foundation established in the beginner chapter. Embrace these new challenges mindfully, always respecting your body's limits.

In this challenge, you were introduced to flow sequences that link poses together smoothly and intentionally. This practice helps build stamina, improve circulation, and enhance overall body awareness. When moving through these poses, try to intentionally deepen your mind-body connection by paying close attention to your breath, sensations, and alignment. Use this awareness to refine your practice and prevent any strain on your body or potential injuries.

Progress takes time and consistency. Celebrate small victories along the way, and be patient with yourself as you explore new challenges and improve your practice.

Chapter 5:

Advanced Level Challenge

What to Expect

Transitioning from intermediate to advanced chair yoga involves a deeper exploration of your practice, focusing on progressing to more challenging poses, fine-tuning technique and alignment, and incorporating resistance for strength training.

This chapter will introduce you to more standing poses that use the chair for support to improve balance, strength, mobility, flexibility, breath awareness, and the mind-body connection.

As you move through these exercises, you'll want to pay close attention to your breath and body alignment in each pose, ensuring proper engagement of muscles and joints. In doing so, you will also improve your mindfulness, allowing you to more readily tune into subtle sensations and cues from your body to deepen your awareness and connection. This is especially important as you move into these challenging poses, as you will need to acknowledge if anything feels too challenging or fast-paced and make adjustments as needed.

You will also incorporate more body-weight resistance into your practice. For example, the first exercise in this chapter, Tricep Dips, uses your body weight to strengthen your arm muscles. It's important to move slowly through these types of exercises so that you can pay close attention to what your body is communicating to you and avoid potential injury. Remember that these exercises are meant to be challenging while still feeling good. If anything feels too strenuous or at all painful, it's okay to stop and reassess.

Advanced Poses for Arms

Tricep Dips

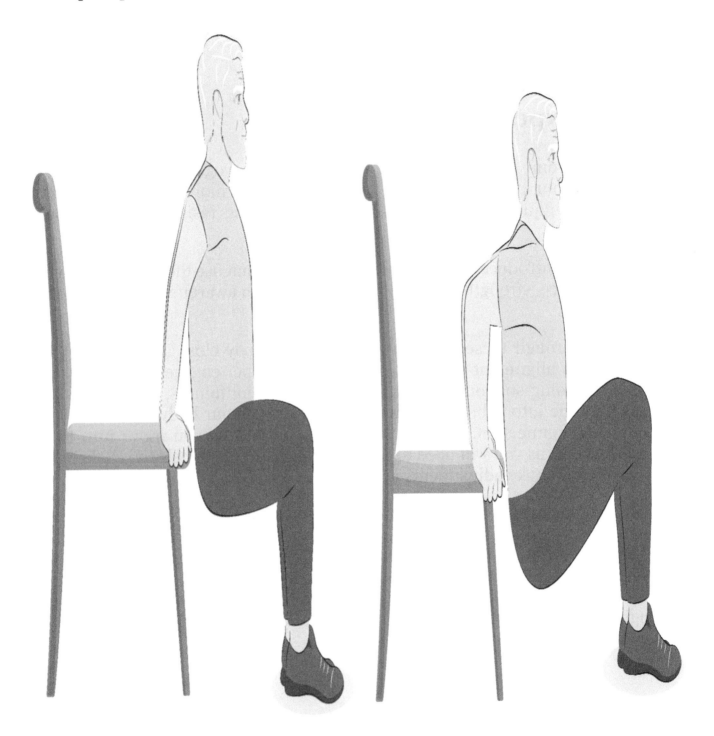

Set up:

- Place your chair against a wall and make sure you have enough room to comfortably move in front of the chair.

Instructions:

- Sit comfortably in your chair and grab the front of the chair's seat with your hands.

- Bring your chest forward until you come off the chair, keeping your arms extended while grabbing onto the seat.

- Shift your torso forward so that your body moves past the edge of the seat.

- Your feet should be slightly in front of your knees, and your knees should be bent.

- On an inhale, slowly bend at the elbows, lowering your upper body toward the floor until your arms are at a 90-degree angle.

- Exhale and extend your arms, raising your upper body back up.

- Perform ten repetitions.

- To release, raise your body back to the chair and bring your palms to your thighs.

Key considerations:

- It's especially important for this exercise that you maintain proper alignment with your legs. Keep your feet flat on the floor and your feet and knees hip-width apart.

- When bending the elbows to lower the torso, the 90-degree angle of your arms should be parallel to the side edges of the chair instead of having your elbows point outward.

- Relax the shoulders and neck. You should feel the exercise in your triceps.

Reverse Plank

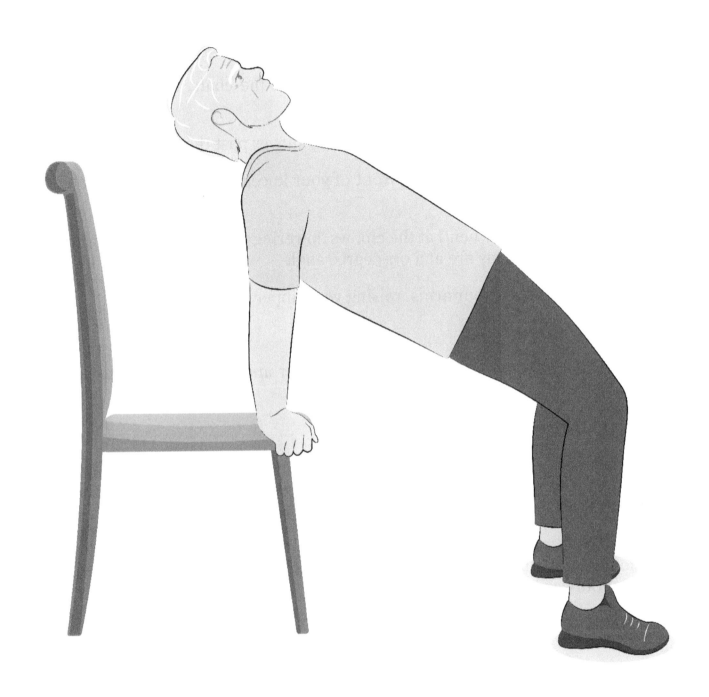

Set up:

- Bring your chair to a comfortable, open area for chair yoga, making sure you have room to move freely in front of your chair.

Instructions:

- Sit comfortably on the edge of your chair and grab the front corners of the chair's seat.

- Walk your feet out a few steps in front of you so that your legs are at about a 140-degree angle with your feet flat on the floor.

- Engage your arm muscles, and on an inhale, slowly lift your hips forward and up until your body is in a straight line from the top of your spine down to your knees.

- Your arms should be perpendicular to the chair with your shoulders directly above your hands, holding the weight of the upper body.

- Keep your knees and ankles aligned to hold the weight of your lower body.

- Make sure your head is in line with your spine to avoid straining your neck.

- Hold here for a few seconds, and then, after an exhale, lower your glutes back down to the chair.

- Repeat this sequence for six repetitions.

Key considerations:

- Maintain a slight bend at the elbows to avoid locking or overextending your arms while in the reverse plank position.

- Keep your core engaged to keep a straight back.

- It's especially important for this exercise that you maintain proper alignment with your legs. Keep your feet shoulder width apart.

Half Moon Pose

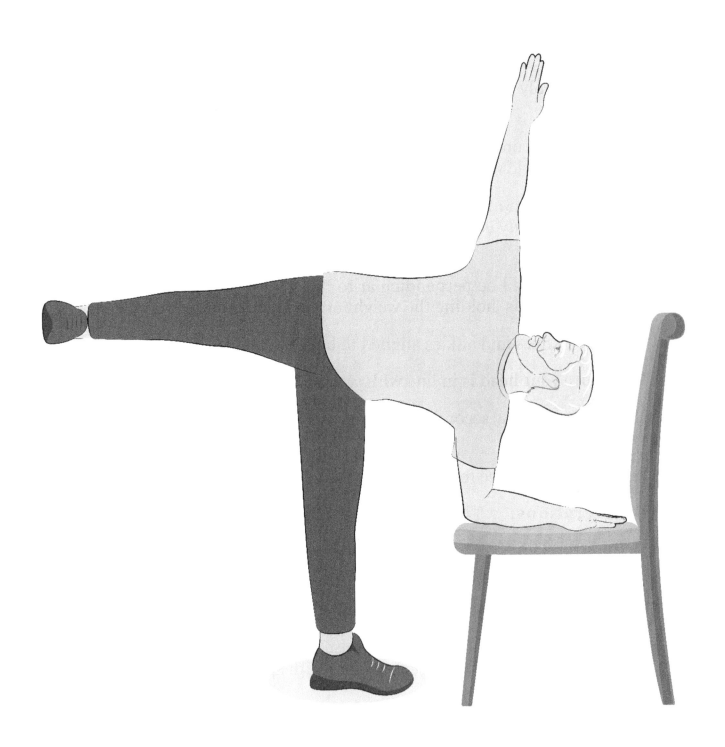

Set up:

- Bring your chair to a comfortable, open area to practice chair yoga, making sure you can fully extend your body in front of the chair.

Instructions:

- Stand a couple of feet away from the seat of your chair. On an inhale, raise your arms over your head. Exhale and lower your forearms onto the seat.

- Inhale and bring your right leg back so that the ball of your foot is making contact with the floor.

- Bend your left knee so that you're in a slight lunge. Exhale.

- Inhale and slowly raise your right foot off the floor, bringing it up until it is parallel to the floor. Exhale and straighten out your left leg.

- Inhale and lift your right arm off the chair, balancing your weight on the left forearm. Exhale. Inhale and raise your right arm, pointing your fingers toward the ceiling.

- Keep your hips in the same position as you twist your upper body and stretch your arm upward. Exhale. Inhale and open up your right hip so that your whole body is facing right.

- Turn your head to look up at your right hand and hold for five deep breaths.

- To come out of the pose, release your arm and neck, bringing the right arm down to meet the left. Rotate your hip to face downward and bring your right leg back down to meet the left. Raise your torso to stand.

- Repeat this sequence once more on the other side.

Key considerations:

- Place your chair against a wall if you're worried about the chair slipping.

- Engage your core to maintain a straight back that's parallel to the floor.

- This pose relies heavily on balance. If you don't feel comfortably stable enough to move directly into the next position change, hold where you are for a few breaths until you feel comfortable moving on.

Upward Facing Dog Pose

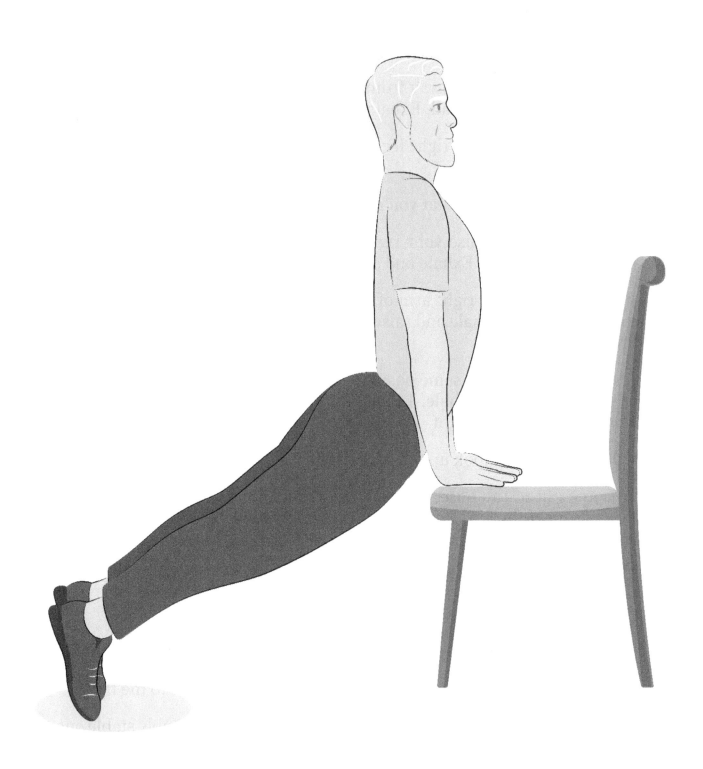

Set up:

- Place your chair in a comfortable and open area to practice chair yoga.

- You can place the chair against a wall if you're worried about it slipping when you lean your body weight on it.

Instructions:

- Stand a couple of feet in front of your chair.

- Bend your torso down toward the chair and grab the edges of the chair's seat.

- Walk your feet back until your body is at about a 45-degree angle from the floor, with your arms straight and supporting your upper body weight.

- The weight of your lower body should be supported by the balls of your feet.

- On an inhale, slowly bring your chest up as you arch your spine. Exhale.

- Inhale and bring your gaze up to the ceiling.

- Hold this pose for 10 deep breaths.

- On an inhale, bring your head back down so you're looking forward and straighten your back.

- Exhale and walk your feet forward.

- Inhale and raise your torso to move back to a standing position.

- Repeat this exercise once through.

Key considerations:

- When arching your back, you should never force the arch past what is comfortable. Make sure your shoulders are dropped, and your neck is relaxed. Think about lengthening the spine as you arch so that you're not compressing the spine.

- Make sure your wrists are in line with your shoulders and your feet are hip-width apart.

Advanced Poses for Neck and Shoulders

Dancing Warrior Pose

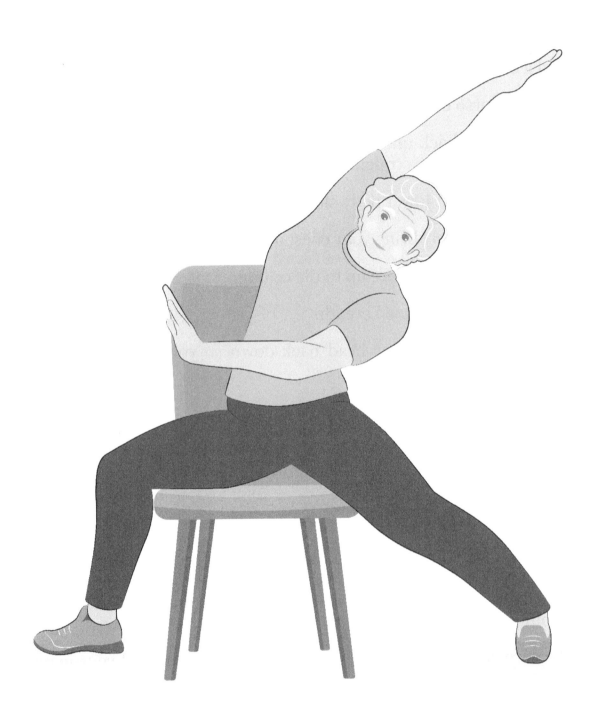

Set up:

- Bring your chair to an open and comfortable area to practice chair yoga and move freely.

Instructions:

- Sit comfortably on the edge of your chair.

- On an inhale, spread your legs into a wide stance with your left leg stretched out to the left and the foot pointed forward.

- Bring your right leg to a 90-degree angle with your toes pointed toward the right. Exhale.

- Inhale and raise your arms straight out to your sides at shoulder level with your palms facing the floor.

- Exhale and bring your gaze to your right hand.

- Inhale and reach your right arm over your head and to the left as you bring your left arm across your torso, reaching to the right and flexing your hand so that your left palm is pointed to the right.

- Bring your head in line with your right arm so that it's tilted to the left.

- Hold this pose for six deep breaths.

- Slowly release from the pose, bringing your arms down and your head to the center, and then bringing your legs into a neutral seated position.

- Repeat this flow on the other side.

Key considerations:

- Think about reaching your neck up in the direction of your upper hand during the pose. This will help you get the most out of the stretch in your neck.

- Make sure your shoulders are dropped, letting your arms reach in opposite directions as you feel the stretch in your shoulders.

Humble Warrior Pose

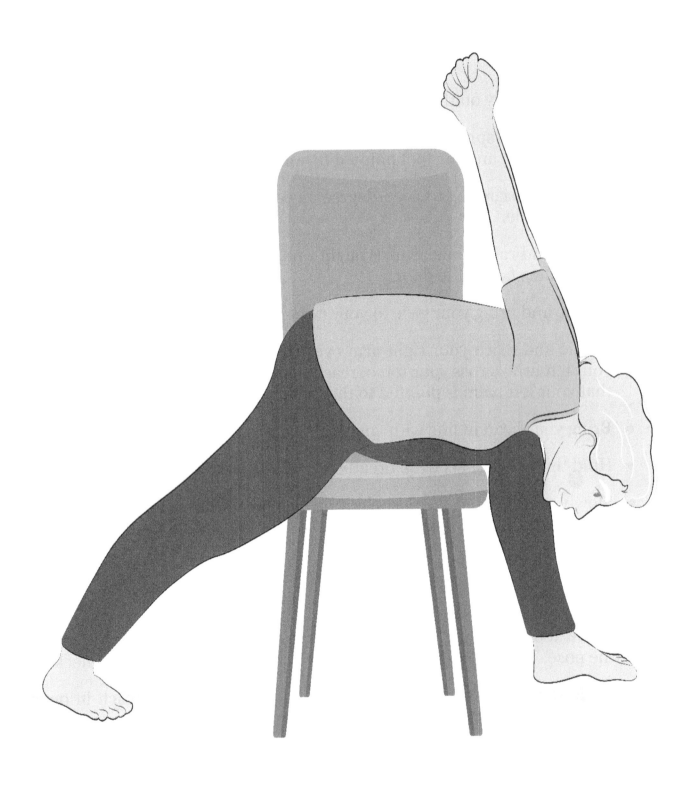

Set up:

- Bring your chair to a comfortable area to practice chair yoga with sufficient room to move freely.

Instructions:

- Sit comfortably toward the edge of your chair.

- Bring your left thigh over the seat of your chair so that your leg is at a 90-degree angle with your foot pointed left.

- Stretch your right leg out to the right with your toes pointed forward.

- On an inhale, bring your hands behind your back and interlace your fingers.

- Exhale and bring your torso down toward your left thigh, keeping a straight back. Your gaze should be toward the floor.

- Inhale and bring your arms up, keeping your fingers intertwined so that your hands are reaching up toward the ceiling.

- Hold this pose for six deep breaths.

- Slowly release yourself from the pose, disengaging your arms first, then bringing your torso up, then bringing your legs together in a neutral seated position.

- Repeat this sequence on the other side.

Key considerations:

- It's okay if you're not able to get your arms perpendicular to the floor in this pose. Reach as far up as you comfortably can and hold the position there.

- Keep a slight bend in the leg which is extended toward the back to avoid straining it.

Sage Marichi Pose

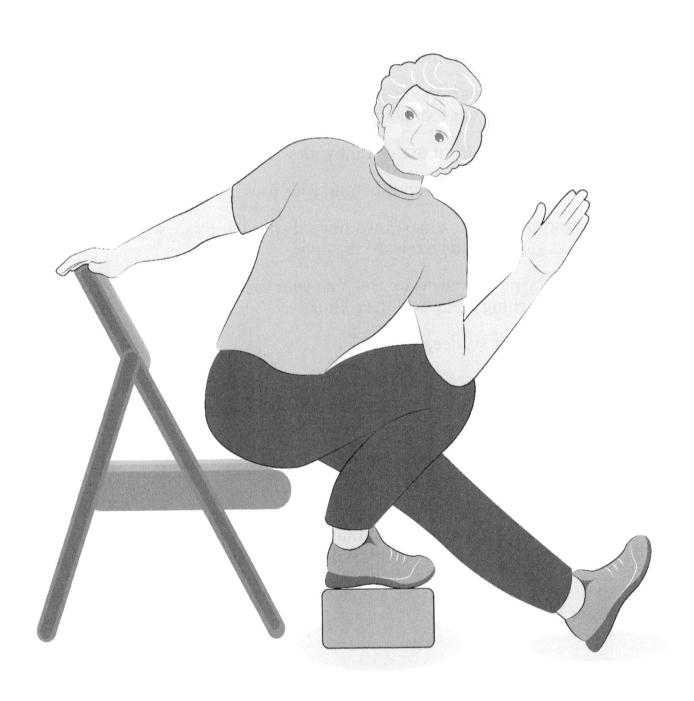

Set up:

- Bring your chair to a comfortable and open area to practice chair yoga.

- Grab a couple of yoga blocks (if you don't own yoga blocks, you can use a stack of books or a couple of rolled-up towels). The height of the yoga blocks or yoga block alternatives should be about a foot. Place the yoga blocks against the front right leg of the chair.

Instructions:

- Sit comfortably toward the edge of your chair.

- On an inhale, reach your legs out in front of you with your heels resting on the floor and your toes flexed upwards.

- Exhale and place your right foot on the yoga blocks.

- Inhale deeply, and on the exhale, twist your torso to the right.

- Grab the back of the chair with your right hand and bring your gaze to the right side.

- Inhale and bring your left elbow to the outside of your right thigh, just above the knee. Your hand should be pointed upwards.

- Exhale and gently press against your thigh with your elbow, deepening the stretch.

- Hold this pose for five deep breaths.

- Release the pose by first disengaging your arms, then untwisting your torso, and then slowly bringing your legs back to a neutral sitting position.

- Repeat this flow on the other side.

Key considerations:

- Make sure your shoulders are dropped throughout this exercise. Engage your core to maintain proper posture and feel the full benefits of the twist stretch.

- Only turn your head as far as feels comfortable for you; don't force the twist stretch in your neck.

Revolved Goddess Pose

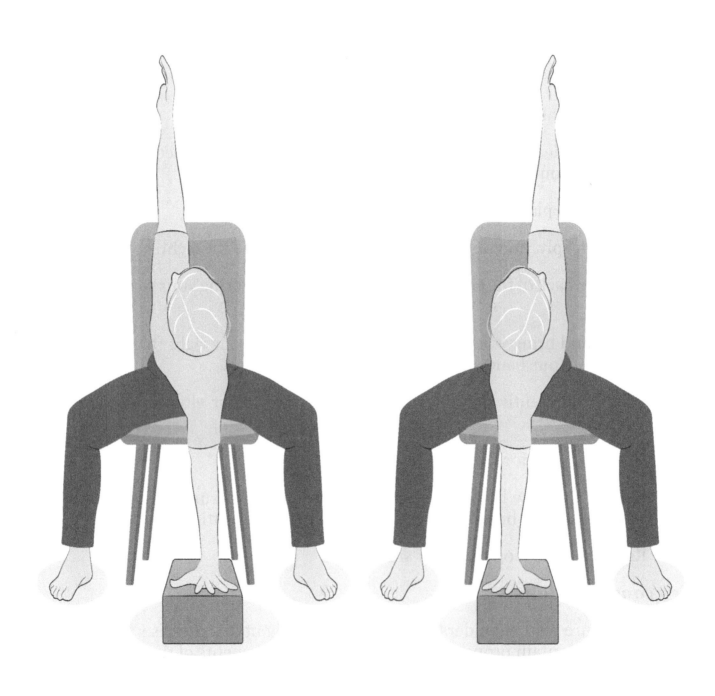

Set up:

- Bring your chair to a comfortable area to practice chair yoga.

- Bring one yoga block or yoga block alternative, and place it about a foot away from the front of your chair.

Instructions:

- Sit comfortably at the edge of your chair.

- On an inhale, spread your legs out wide, with your toes pointed outward. Exhale.

- Inhale and engage your core while lengthening your spine.

- Exhale and slowly bend at the hips, bringing your torso forward and down.

- Bring your arms down so that your palms are resting on the yoga block in front of you.

- Inhale and reach your right arm up with your fingers pointed toward the ceiling as you twist your body to the right. Exhale.

- Inhale and bring your gaze up to your right fingertips.

- Hold this pose for six deep breaths.

- Slowly release the pose by untwisting your upper body, then bring your right arm back down to meet the left arm on an exhale.

- Keeping the position of your legs, repeat this sequence on the other side.

- Fully release at the end by lifting your torso upright and then bringing your legs back to the starting position in front of the chair.

Key considerations:

- Make sure your knees are in line with your ankles throughout this exercise.

- Instead of relying on your arm to hold up your upper body, engage your core to carry some of the weight so that you're maintaining proper alignment in your spine while in the pose.

Advanced Poses for Chest and Back

Crescent Lunge

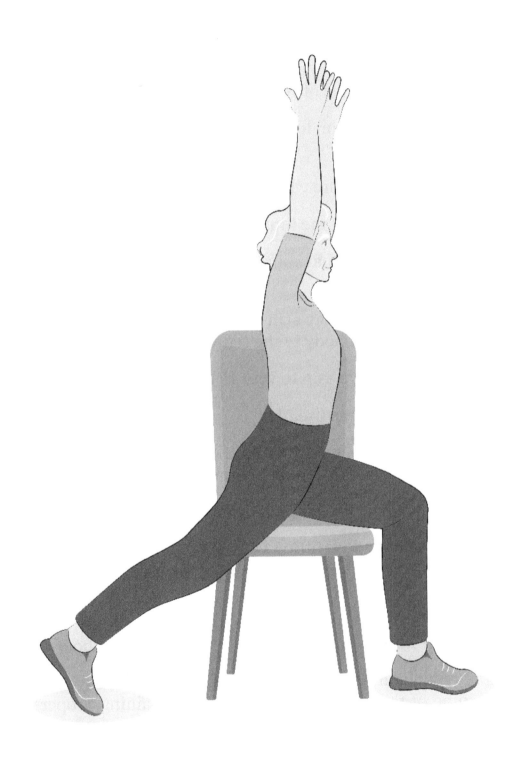

Set up:

- Place your chair in your designated chair yoga area, making sure that you have sufficient room to move freely without bumping into anything.

Instructions:

- Sit comfortably on the edge of your chair and rotate your body so that you're facing the left.

- Keep your left thigh resting across the seat of the chair with your leg bent at a 90-degree angle and your left foot facing the left.

- Let your right leg hang from the chair at a 90-degree angle with your knee and the ball of your foot resting on the floor.

- Slowly extend your right leg behind you so that the leg comes to about a 140-degree angle.

- On an inhale, reach your arms over your head with your palms facing each other and your fingertips pointed toward the ceiling.

- Feel your upper body lengthen as it extends upward.

- Hold here for six deep breaths.

- Slowly come out of the pose by first releasing your arms, then bringing your right leg forward so that it returns to its previous 90-degree angle.

- Shift your weight so that you're firmly planted on your chair, turn so you're facing forward on the chair, and bring your legs up to a neutral seated position.

- Flow into the same sequence on the other side.

Key considerations:

- To help with balance, you can bring your arms out to your sides instead of directly over your head. Make sure your shoulders are dropped and your arms are shoulder-height.

- Keep your core engaged to maintain your posture; ensure your spine is straight and your head is resting gently on top of your shoulders, without slouching or leaning backward or forward.

Wide Stance Fold

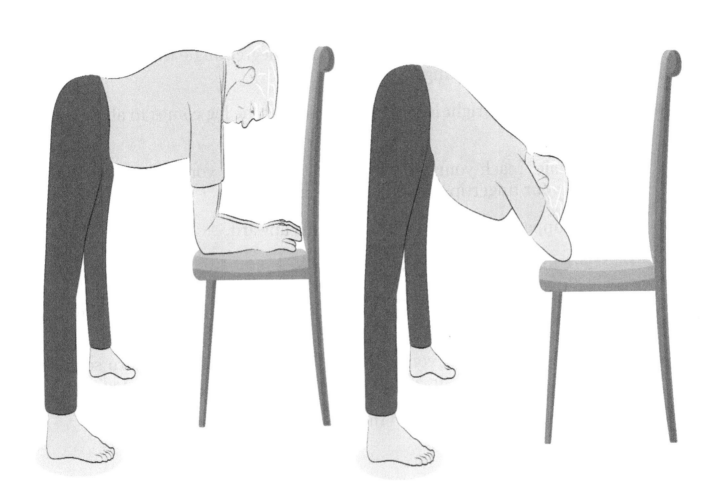

Set up:

- Bring your chair to a comfortable area to practice chair yoga, making sure you have sufficient room to move in front of the chair.

- You can also place the chair against a wall if you're concerned about it slipping when you lean into it.

Instructions:

- Stand a few feet away from your chair, facing the front.

- Widen your stance so that your feet are wider than the chair's legs, with your toes still facing forward.

- Inhale and roll your shoulders back, bringing your gaze upward slightly.

- Feel your chest open up as you do so.

- Exhale and hinge at the hips, bringing your torso down toward the seat of the chair while maintaining a straight back.

- Rest your forearms on the seat of the chair.

- Inhale and walk your feet out, slightly widening your stance.

- From here, gently begin to rock your weight forward and then backward.

- Slow to a halt and fold your forearms over each other at the edge of the chair.

- Place your head on your crossed arms, and feel the stretch gently deepen.

- Feel your spine decompress and hold here for three deep breaths.

- To release, bring your palms together on the seat of the chair. Slowly raise your torso to a standing position and bring your legs together.

Key considerations:

- When positioning your legs in the wide standing stance, go with what feels comfortable for you instead of forcing a stance that feels too broad.

- Maintain a slight bend in the knees and elbows to avoid locking or overextending the joints.

Side Bend

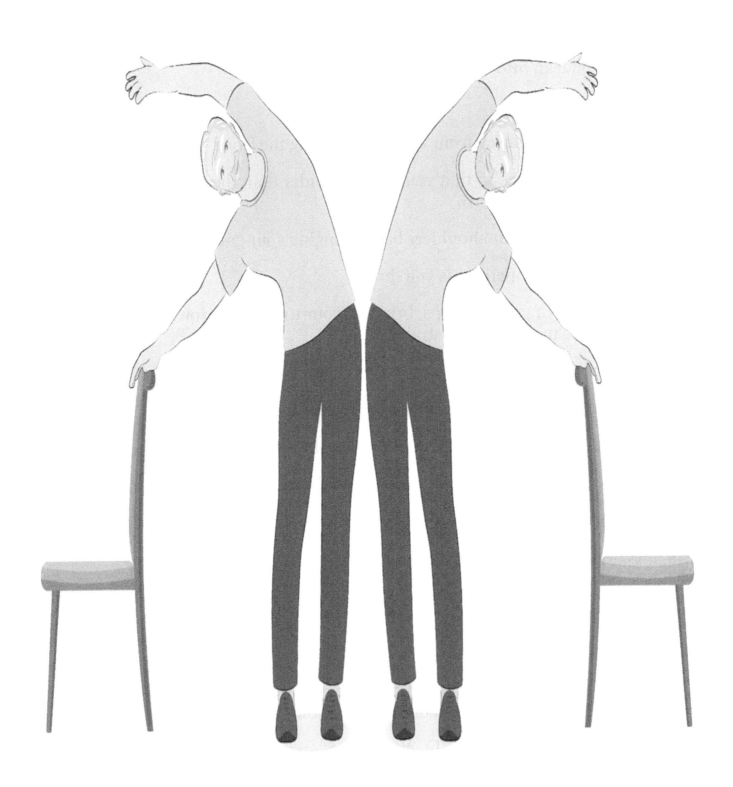

Set up:

- Place your chair in a comfortable, open area to practice chair yoga, ensuring you have enough room to move while standing behind it.

Instructions:

- Stand arm's length away from the back of your chair.

- Bring your right palm to the back of the chair.

- Raise your left arm straight out to the side, at shoulder height.

- On an inhale, raise your left arm toward the ceiling.

- On an exhale, gently press against the chair with your right hand as you move your hips to the left.

- Reach your left arm over your head and toward the chair, and let your upper body follow in this stretch.

- Hold this pose for six deep breaths.

- On an exhale, bring your left arm back up, over your head, and down to your side.

- Let your torso follow until you're in an upright position.

- Turn around and repeat this sequence on the other side.

Key considerations:

- When bending the torso and raising the arm toward the chair, think about lengthening through the spine, the top of the head, and the arm as you stretch toward the chair. This will help keep your posture tall and prevent any compression.

- Keep your head in line with your neck to avoid straining it as you tilt your upper body to one side.

Twist Pose

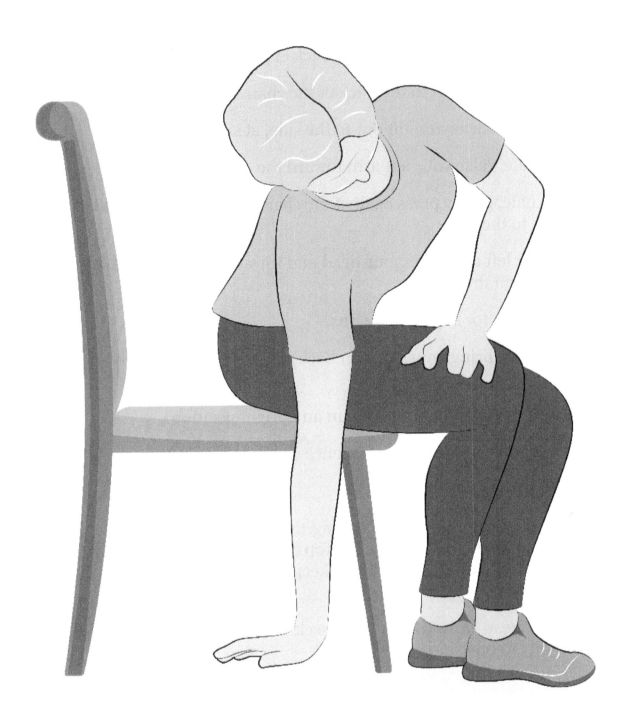

Set up:

- Bring your chair to a comfortable area to practice chair yoga, making sure that you have enough room to move freely while seated.

Instructions:

- Sit comfortably in your chair with your palms resting on your thighs.

- On an inhale, bring your left foot around in front of your right foot with the soles of both feet resting on the floor.

- Exhale and place your left palm on the outer right thigh, just above the knee.

- Lower your upper body to the right side and place your right hand on the floor to the right side of your chair so that your palm is on the floor and your fingers are pointed backward.

- Your head and neck should be in line with the position of your shoulders.

- Gently press your left palm against your right leg and deepen the stretch.

- Stay here for six full breaths.

- Slowly release by disengaging your left arm, then slowly bringing your torso upright to a sitting posture, then untwisting your feet and coming back to a neutral seated position.

- Repeat this sequence on the other side.

Key considerations:

- Only twist as far as feels comfortable for you. Don't force the stretch. Make sure your shoulders are dropped, and your core is engaged to help maintain proper posture throughout the flow.

- If you are struggling to place your palm on the floor, place a stack of books next to you and try to place your palm on these. Gradually, reduce the number of books to eventually place your palm on the floor.

Advanced Poses for Abs

Rows

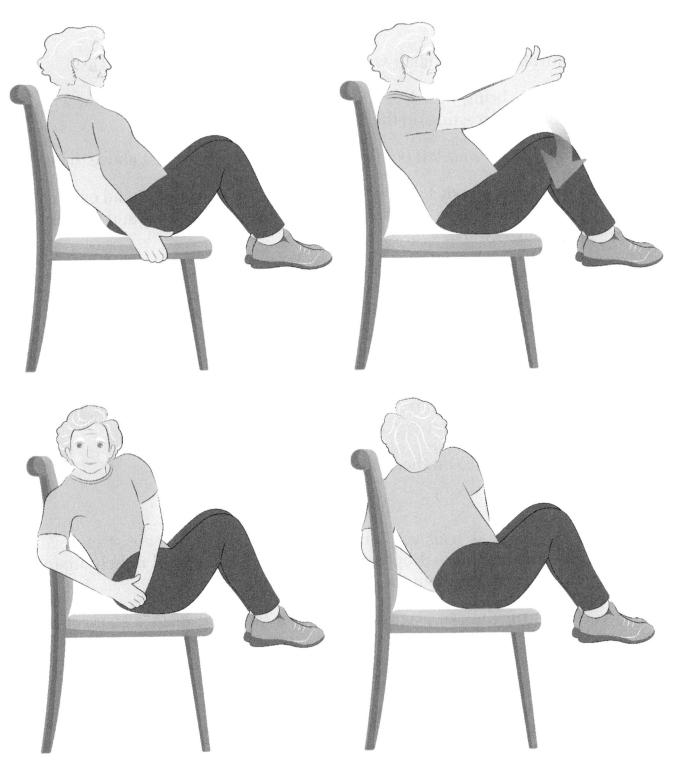

Set up:

- Bring your chair to a comfortable area to practice chair yoga, making sure you have enough room to move freely.

Instructions:

- Sit comfortably toward the edge of your chair and grab the sides of the chair's seat with your hands.

- Engage your core and lean your torso back a bit so that your shoulders are touching the back of the chair without leaning your weight into it.

- Bring your legs up so that they're at about a 90-degree angle, hovering above the floor.

- Slowly release your hands from the chair, extending them out to the front.

- Hold here for three deep breaths, feeling yourself get accustomed to this pose.

- Bring your hands up by your core, and slowly bring them to your right side and then to your left side, as if you were rowing a boat.

- Repeat this rowing pattern 10 times.

- To release, slowly bring your arms to a stop, and on an exhale, slowly drop your arms down, followed by your legs.

Key considerations:

- Take your time when you're moving through the steps for this pose, as you may need to take some additional time to get used to the balance aspect of these movements.

- Make sure to also remember to breathe. If you're taking a slower pace with the rowing motion, you can try inhaling as you row to one side and exhaling as you bring your arms over to row on the other side. If you're going with a quicker pace, you can try inhaling as you row right and left one time and then exhaling as you row right and left in the next repetition.

Flutter Kicks

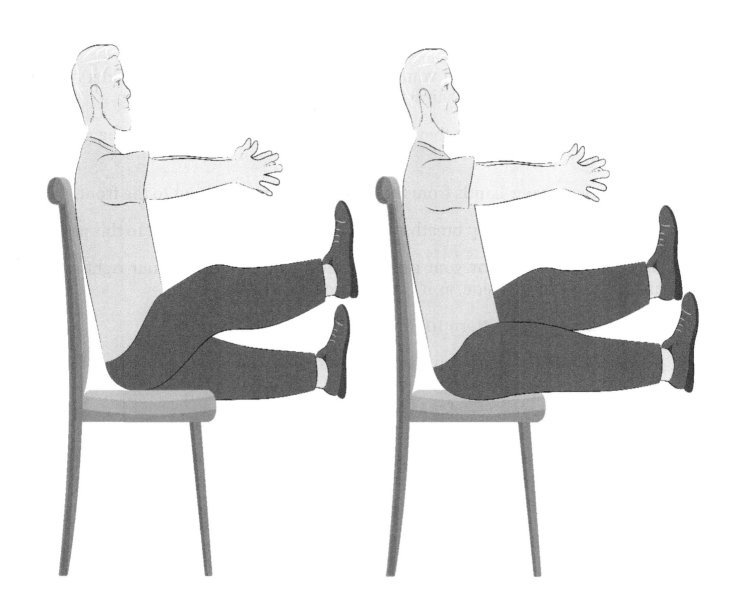

Set up:

- Bring your chair to a comfortable space to practice chair yoga, making sure that you have sufficient room to extend your legs fully while seated.

Instructions:

- Sit comfortably in your chair with your palms resting on your thighs.

- On an inhale, extend your legs in front of you, raising your feet off the floor.

- Exhale and reach your arms out in front of you so that they're parallel to your legs, with your palms facing each other.

- On an inhale, move your right leg gently up while keeping your other leg held up in the air.

- Exhale and lower the right leg back to meet the left leg.

- Inhale again and move your left leg gently up while keeping your other leg held up in the air.

- Exhale and lower the left leg back to meet the right leg.

- Continue fluttering your legs for about twenty seconds, remembering to breathe throughout.

- To release, slowly lower your feet back down to the floor and your palms back down to your thighs.

Key considerations:

- The flutter kicks should be performed at a relatively quick pace; however, you can build up to this speed. Especially if it's your first time performing this exercise, you'll want to gradually increase your pace as you get used to the motions and the balance that the exercise requires.

- Your movements during this exercise should be fluid. Allowing your breath to guide you will help you with this.

Oblique Crunches

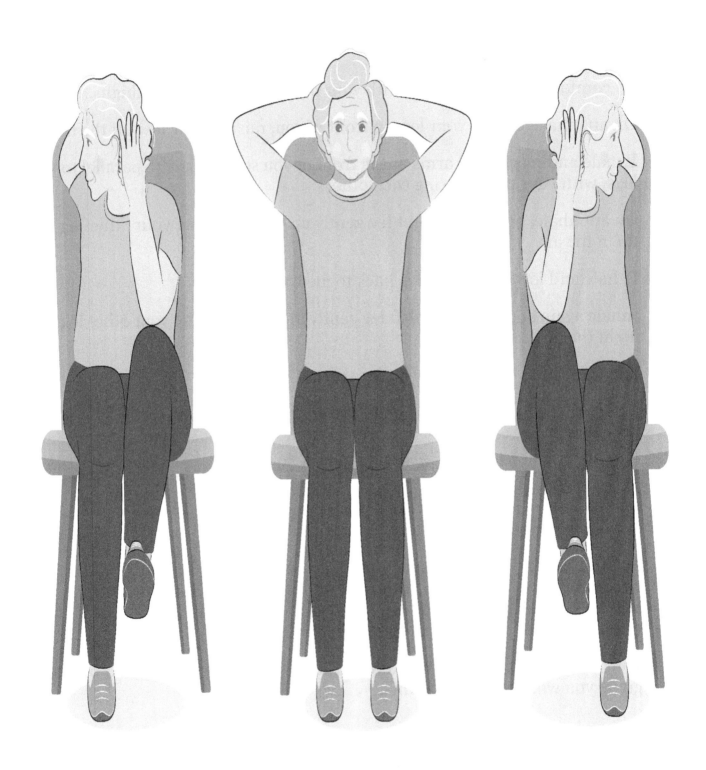

Set up:

- Bring your chair to a comfortable and open area to practice chair yoga. Make sure you have sufficient room to move comfortably without hitting anything.

Instructions:

- Sit comfortably toward the edge of your chair.

- Walk your feet out so that your legs are at about a 140-degree angle.

- On an inhale, bring your palms to the back of your head with your elbow pointed out to the sides.

- Exhale and raise your left knee while bringing your left elbow down to meet each other.

- Touch the knee and the elbow together and hold here for a second before releasing back to the starting position on an inhale.

- Repeat this motion for 10 repetitions on this side before slowing down to a stop and releasing back to the starting position.

- After the last repetition, move to the other side and repeat the same sequence for 10 repetitions.

- To release, place your foot back on the floor and then place your hands in your lap.

Key considerations:

- Keep your shoulders loose and your neck straight and relaxed throughout the exercise.

- Your movements during this exercise should be fluid. Allowing your breath to guide you will help you with this.

Dolphin Plank

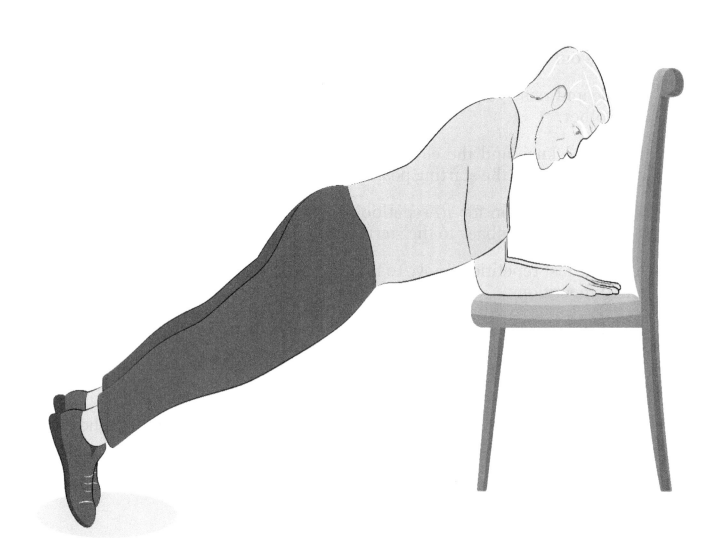

Set up:

- Place your chair against a wall, and make sure you have enough room to fully extend your body in front of the chair.

Instructions:

- Stand a couple of feet away from your chair.

- Slowly bend at the hips, lowering your torso toward the seat, and rest your forearms on the seat with your fingers pointed toward the back of the chair.

- Walk your feet back until your body is straight.

- Your weight should be resting on your forearms and the balls of your feet.

- Make sure that you keep you core muscles engaged to keep a straight back and keep your head in line with your spine to avoid straining your neck.

- Hold this position for ten deep breaths.

- To release, slowly walk your feet forward and then raise your torso to come back to a standing position.

- Repeat this exercise once through.

Key considerations:

- While in the dolphin plank pose, engage your core and keep your hips tucked to maintain a straight, aligned position.

- With many abdominal exercises, people tend to hold their breath or restrict their breathing. This is especially true when you are in a position that works your abs. To make sure that you're breathing properly, bring your attention to your rib cage. As you inhale, you should be able to feel and see your rib cage expanding. As you exhale, you should feel and see it contract.

Advanced Poses for Legs

Dancer's Pose

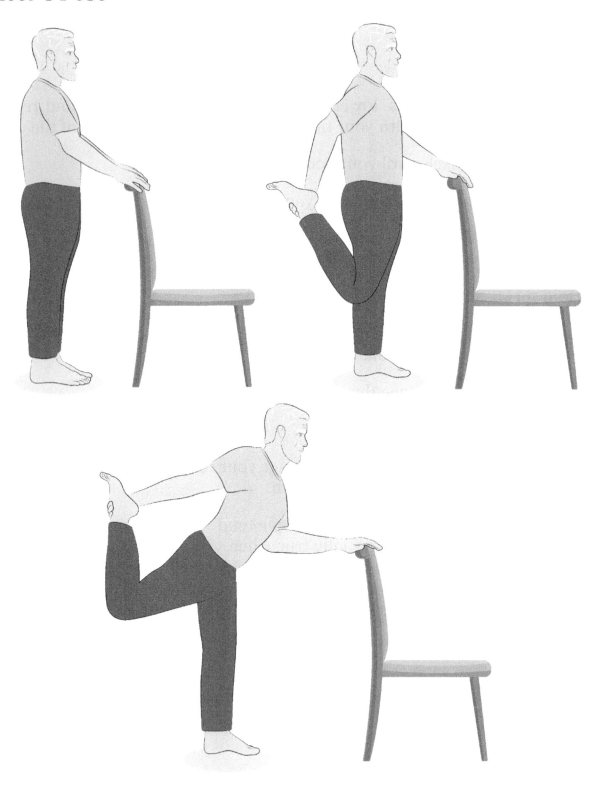

Set up:

- Bring your chair to an open, comfortable area for chair yoga. Check that you have plenty of room to move behind your chair without hitting anything.

Instructions:

- Stand behind your chair and grab onto the back of the chair.

- Bending at the knee, bring your right foot up toward your glutes.

- Hold onto your foot with your right hand.

- Gently press your foot toward your body.

- Slowly bring your torso forward while maintaining your hold on your right foot with the right hand and the back of the chair with your left hand.

- Maintain a straight back and engage your core as you bend forward.

- Hold this pose for five deep breaths.

- Slowly return to an upright position and release your leg back down.

- Repeat this sequence with the other leg.

Key considerations:

- If you aren't able to grab your foot, you can use a strap or a belt to loop around your foot.

- Only bend forward in this pose, however far it feels comfortable for you. You don't want to force the stretch here; move slowly and pay attention to how your body feels. You should feel a nice stretch in your quad.

Rock the Baby

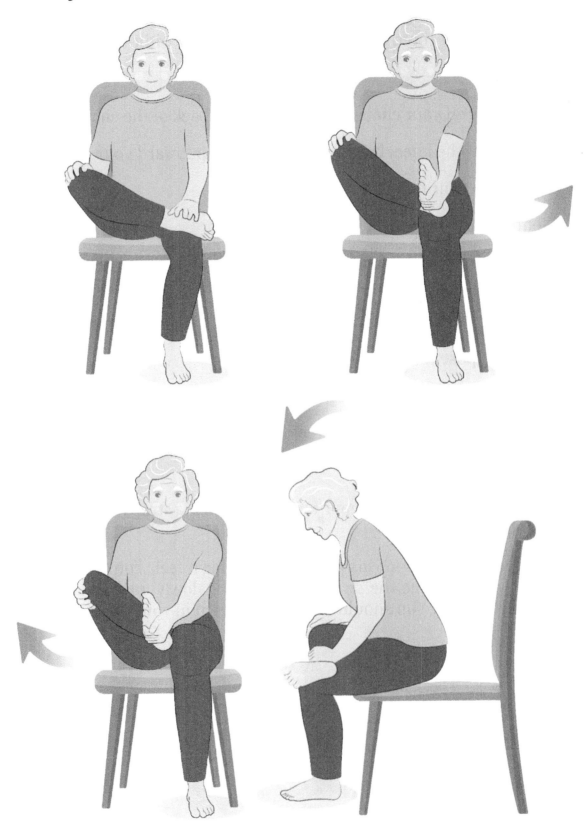

Set up:

- Bring your chair to your designated chair yoga space, making sure that you have enough room to comfortably move.

Instructions:

- Sit comfortably in your chair, and lift your right leg up, maintaining the bend at the knee and place your right foot on your left knee.

- Bring your left hand to your right foot and your right hand to your right knee.

- Rotate your right hip out so that you can bring your shin into a diagonal position.

- Slowly release your right foot from your left knee, lifting it up slightly and start to rock your leg from side to side, feeling the motion loosen up your right hip joint.

- Rock for about thirty seconds, remembering to breathe throughout.

- From here, lower your right ankle over your left thigh, just above the knee.

- Gently lower your right knee down so that your shin is parallel to the floor.

- Slowly bend forward at the waist until you feel a nice stretch in your outer right hip. Hold here for four deep breaths.

- On an inhale, bring your torso back upright.

- On an exhale, gently release your right leg back down to a neutral seated position.

- Repeat this sequence with your left leg.

Key considerations:

- Move slowly through this exercise as it works for your flexibility and mobility. You want to be sure that everything feels comfortable on the joints before continuing with the flow.

- Make sure to move through this exercise in a controlled manner and to breathe throughout to prevent any potential lightheadedness.

Hamstring Stretch

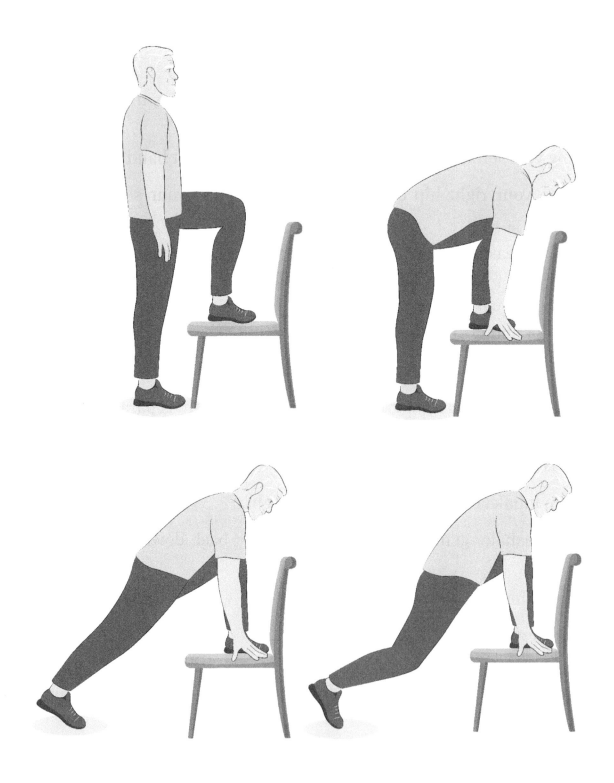

Set up:

- Bring your chair to a comfortable, open area to practice chair yoga, and make sure that you have plenty of room to move in front of your chair. You can also place your chair against a wall if you're concerned about the chair slipping when you lean your weight into it.

Instructions:

- Stand a few feet away from your chair and place your left foot on the chair.

- Place your palms on the seat of the chair on either side of your foot.

- Move your right leg back to feel a stretch in your hamstring and hip flexors.

- Keep your spine straight, your shoulders down and back, and your gaze forward. Hold this pose for four deep breaths.

- Gently bend your right knee slightly to feel a stretch in your quad as well.

- Bring your right foot forward on the floor a bit, shifting your weight back slightly so that the sole of your right foot is flat on the floor and most of your weight is resting on it. As you do so, your left leg will straighten out a bit, and your foot will come off the chair so that only your heel is resting on the seat.

- Make sure your hips are square (both pointed forward) and your back is straight and feel the stretch in your left hamstring. Hold this pose for four deep breaths.

- Slowly bring your left leg back to the floor and come into a neutral standing position before moving into the same sequence with the other leg.

Key considerations:

- In the first part of the flow, maintain a slight bend in your back leg to avoid overextending or locking the knee. You can also increase the bend in the back leg from the start if it feels more comfortable for you.

- During the second part of the flow, maintain a bend in your lifted leg. Bend as much as you'd like, but make sure that you can still feel the stretch. You can also keep a straighter leg and remove your hands from the seat of the chair, but make sure you're comfortable with the balance aspect of this move.

Side Angle Pose

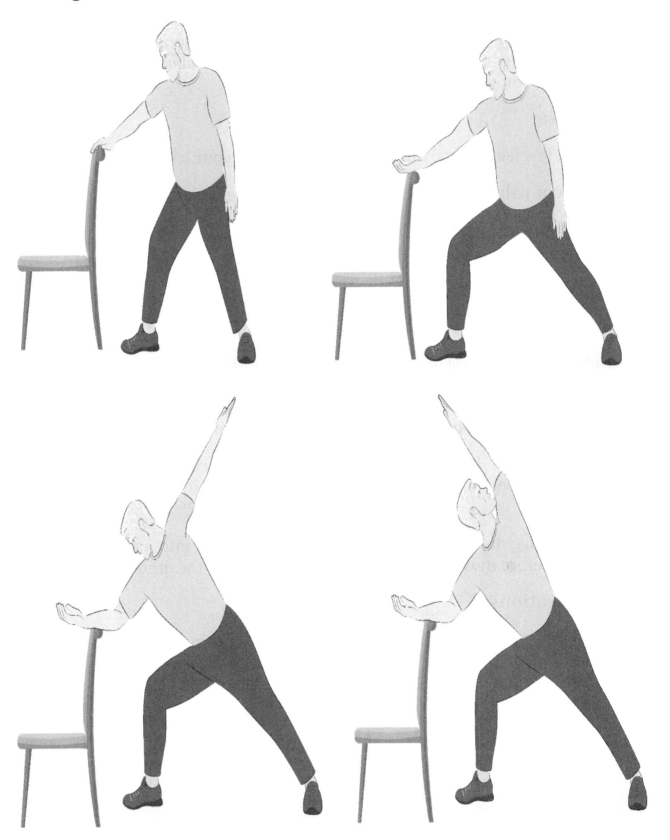

Set up:

- Bring your chair to a comfortable, open area to practice chair yoga. Check that you have plenty of room to move freely behind your chair.

Instructions:

- Stand behind your chair and bring your right hand to the back of the chair.

- Bring your right foot forward so that your toes are pointed toward the chair and your knee is slightly bent.

- Bring your left foot back so that your toes are pointed slightly outward toward the left and your leg is straight.

- Rotate the arm so that your palm is facing upward.

- Slide your right arm forward so that your forearm is resting on the back of the chair.

- On an inhale, engage your core, circle your left arm up and over your head, and stretch your fingertips to your right. Exhale.

- On an inhale, open your chest as you bring your left shoulder slightly back.

- Bring your gaze up toward the crook of your left elbow.

- Hold this position for six deep breaths.

- Release the pose by bringing your gaze forward, disengaging the arms, and then coming to a standing position.

- Turn around and flow straight into the same exercise on the other side.

Key considerations:

- When you're bending your forward leg, make sure your knee is over your ankle. This is as far as you need to take the bend at the knee.

- Only stretch your arm as far as is comfortable for you. When doing so, make sure to keep your spine straight, your shoulders relaxed and dropped, and your head and neck aligned with your spine.

Weekly Routine

Week 1

Day 1
- Begin with **Tricep Dips** (page 104) for 10 reps.
- Flow directly into **Dancing Warrior Pose** (page 112), holding for six breaths per side.
- Flow directly into **Flutter Kicks** (page 130) for 20 seconds.

Day 2
- Begin with **Dancer's Pose** (page 136), holding for five breaths per side.
- Move directly into **Side Angle Pose** (page 142), holding six breaths per side.
- From here, flow straight into **Side Bends** (page 124) for six breaths per side.

Week 2

Day 1
- Begin with **Dolphin Plank** (page 134) for 10 breaths.
- Release into standing and flow directly into **Wide Stance Fold** (page 122) for three reps per side.
- From here, move straight into **Hamstring Stretch** (page 140) for four breaths in the first position, then four breaths in the second position. Repeat the sequence once more on the other side.

Day 2
- Begin with **Reverse Plank** (page 106) for six reps.
- Flow directly into **Crescent Lunge** (page 120) for six breaths per side.
- From here, move straight into **Revolved Goddess Pose** (page 118) for six breaths per side.

Day 3
- Begin with **Sage Marichi Pose** (page 116), holding for five breaths per side.

- Flow straight into **Twist Pose** (page 126), holding for six breaths per side.

- Finish out by flowing into **Rock the Baby** (page 138) for 30 seconds, then flowing into the stretch position for four breaths. Repeat this sequence on the other side.

Week 3

Day 1

- Start with **Oblique Crunches** (page 132), performing 10 reps per side.

- Flow straight into **Humble Warrior Pose** (page 114), holding for six breaths per side.

- From here, flow into **Crescent Lunge** (page 120) for six breaths per side.

- Move directly from here into **Twist Pose** (page 126), holding for six breaths per side.

Day 2

- Begin with **Half Moon Pose** (page 108), holding for five breaths per side.

- Come up directly into the **Hamstring Stretch** (page 140), holding for four breaths in the first position, then four breaths in the second position. Repeat the sequence on the other side.

- Come to a sitting position and move into **Row** (page 128) for 10 reps.

- Flow straight into **Dancing Warrior Pose** (page 112), holding for six breaths per side.

Day 3

- Start with the **Upward Facing Dog Pose** (page 110), holding for 10 breaths.

- Flow directly into **Dolphin Plank** (page 134), holding for 10 breaths.

- Come up and move behind your chair. Move into **Side Bends** (page 124) for six breaths per side.

- From here, flow into **Dancer's Pose** (page 136), holding for five breaths per side.

Day 4

- Start with **Half Moon Pose** (page 108) for five breaths per side.

- Flow straight into **Wide Stance Fold** (page 122) for three reps per side.

- Sit in your chair and move into **Flutter Kicks** (page 130) for 20 seconds.

- From here, flow into **Rock the Baby** (page 138) for 30 seconds, then flow into the stretch position for four breaths. Repeat on the other side.

Week 4

Day 1

- Start with a **Side Angle Pose** (page 142) for six breaths per side.

- Come around to the front of your chair and move into **Tricep Dips** (page 104) for 10 reps.

- Come out of the exercise into a seated position and move into **Humble Warrior Pose** (page 114) for six breaths per side.

- Flow straight into **Reverse Plank** (page 106) for six reps.

Day 2

- Start with **Twist Pose** (page 104) for six breaths per side.

- Move directly into **Rows** (page 128) for 10 reps.

- From here, flow into the **Revolved Goddess Pose** (page 118) for six breaths per side.

- Flow directly into **Crescent Lunge** (page 120), holding for six breaths per side.

Day 3

- Start with **Sage Marichi Pose** (page 116) for five breaths per side.

- Flow into **Oblique Crunches** (page 132) for 10 reps per side.

- Come to standing and move into the **Upward Facing Dog Pose** (page 110), holding for 10 breaths.

- From here, flow into **Hamstring Stretch** (page 140) for four breaths in the first position, then four in the second position. Repeat on the other side.

Day 4

- Start with **Tricep Dips** (page 104) for 10 reps.

- Finish in a seated position and flow into **Dancing Warrior Pose** (page 112) for six breaths per side.

- Flow into **Reverse Plank** (page 106), performing six reps.

- Finish out by flowing into **Rows** (page 128) for 10 reps.

Key Takeaways

Moving into the advanced 28-day chair yoga challenge marks a significant milestone in your practice. You're now able to flow into more challenging and dynamic poses, hold poses for longer, make transitions more seamlessly, and experience a greater sense of strength, mobility, balance, and flexibility.

Advanced chair yoga also requires a heightened level of focus and concentration, leading to a deeper awareness of your body, breath, and mental state. This increased awareness can enhance your overall well-being and mindfulness, both on and off the mat.

Now is a great time to look back to where you were at the beginning of your chair yoga journey and how far you've come.

Chapter 6:

Nutrition and Lifestyle Tips

A Balanced Diet

The core principles of chair yoga embrace holistic health; with this in mind, there are other factors outside of chair yoga that you should take into consideration to reach your goals.

A balanced diet is crucial for maintaining overall health and well-being. It provides the necessary nutrients, vitamins, and minerals that your body needs to function at its best. To create a balanced diet, include a variety of ingredients from all food groups, including fruits, vegetables, whole grains, lean proteins, and healthy fats.

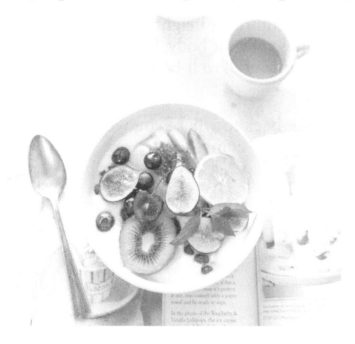

Following a balanced diet also involves being mindful of portion sizes and choosing foods rich in vitamins and nutrients.

It's also essential to stay hydrated by drinking plenty of water throughout the day, as water helps regulate body temperature, aids in digestion, and helps your organs function properly.

Additionally, getting enough rest is necessary for your body to repair and rejuvenate. Aim for 7–9 hours of sleep per night to ensure you're well-rested and ready to tackle the day ahead.

Dehydration, poor diet, and diminished sleep quality will all prevent you from performing your best, whether it's physical activity like chair yoga, mental clarity and focus like job performance, or emotional energy like navigating relationships.

Intermittent Fasting

Intermittent fasting is a dietary approach that alternates between periods of eating and fasting. It stands out from other diets because, rather than providing a strict diet regimen, it leaves you with the flexibility to tailor meals to your dietary needs and preferences. It works by targeting the time of day that you eat. There are several methods of intermittent fasting, but the most common ones involve daily 16-hour fasts or fasting for 24 hours once or twice per week.

Start with a 12-hour overnight fast, and gradually add one hour to the fast per week until you reach 16 hours.

During fasting periods, you consume little to no calories. However, you can drink water, coffee, tea, and other naturally non-caloric beverages. The idea behind intermittent fasting is to change your body's hormone levels to make stored body fat more accessible for energy. This can lead to weight loss and other health benefits, such as improved insulin sensitivity, improved metabolic health, longevity, and reduced inflammation.

Intermittent fasting can be incorporated into a chair yoga practice by timing your eating window around your yoga sessions. For example, you could practice chair yoga during your fasting period and break your fast with a nutritious meal afterward. This can help maximize the benefits of both practices and promote overall well-being.

Incorporating Physical Activity Outside of Chair Yoga

In addition to chair yoga, it's important to incorporate other forms of physical activity into your routine to maintain a healthy, active lifestyle. This can include activities such as walking, cycling, dancing, swimming, or strength training.

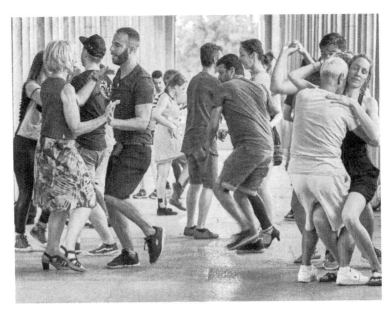

Finding physical activities you genuinely enjoy makes all the difference in the effectiveness of the activity in your life. When you love what you do, it goes from being something that you have to do to something that you look forward to every day. Aim to do something physical every day, whether it's walking, dancing, or chair yoga.

Remember to listen to your body and consult with a healthcare professional before starting any new exercise regimen, especially if you have any underlying health conditions.

Key Takeaways

Incorporate a balanced diet by focusing on foods that are rich in nutrients like fruits, vegetables, whole grains, lean proteins, and healthy fats. Practice mindful eating by paying attention to hunger and fullness cues and savoring each bite.

You may want to give intermittent fasting a try, as it is a way to improve metabolic health, thus promoting weight loss. Remember that it'll take time for your body to adjust to intermittent fasting, so start gradually and listen to your body's cues.

Physical activity is another essential factor in weight loss and overall well-being. Aim for regular exercise, and gradually increase the intensity and duration of your workouts as your fitness level improves. Choose activities that you enjoy, and that fit your lifestyle, making it easier to stick with them in the long term.

Conclusion

Now that you've finished reading this book, you are equipped with all the tools needed to make a real change in your life and start embracing and prioritizing your health and well-being. Your commitment to the 28-day challenge is truly remarkable, and hopefully, it is just the start of your journey toward improving your holistic health.

Getting this far is a reflection of your commitment, and now is a great time to celebrate your progress. If you keep a yoga journal, it's often beneficial to go back and read old passages to reflect on where you were, both mentally and physically, at the start of your journey, to see how you've progressed and maintained your commitment over time, and to congratulate yourself on the wins you've achieved in the process.

The 28-day challenge is meant to kickstart your chair yoga routine and get you ready to start living a more healthy, mindful, and active lifestyle. To sustain the momentum you've created throughout the challenge, remember to find enjoyment in whatever physical activity you do. To continue with chair yoga, you may want to change up the poses in your routine now and then to keep things engaging and to continue challenging yourself.

Establishing a regular schedule for your chair yoga practice and other physical activities can help turn these exercises into habits, making them easier and more enjoyable to maintain over time.

It's also beneficial to share your passions with others. Try joining a chair yoga class or finding a community of like-minded individuals who can provide support and encouragement. Sharing your journey with others can make the process more enjoyable and motivating.

Continue to keep track of your progress. As you reach more of your goals, you'll want to keep challenging yourself to meet new ones. Setting new goals will help you define why you want to practice chair yoga or other physical activities.

Remember that this is an ongoing journey toward improved physical and mental health. Staying motivated to continue through consistent practice will keep pushing you forward. It is never too late to make a change in your life. Now is your time!

References

Arms to side rotations chair. (n.d.a.). Tummee. https://www.tummee.com/yoga-poses/arms-to-side-rotations-chair

Bartlett, D. (2019). *Dancing warrior pose*. Human Kinetics. https://us.humankinetics.com/blogs/excerpt/dancing-warrior-pose#:~:text=Straddle%20the%20seat%20of%20a,the%20front%20and%20the%20back.

Benefits of Healthy Eating. (2021, May 16). CDC. https://www.cdc.gov/nutrition/resources-publications/benefits-of-healthy-eating.html

Better sleep: Why it's important for your health and tips to sleep soundly. (2023, March 15). UC Davis Health. https://health.ucdavis.edu/blog/cultivating-health/better-sleep-why-its-important-for-your-health-and-tips-to-sleep-soundly/2023/03

Capritto, A. (2021, February 17). *How to engage your core*. VeryWell Fit. https://www.verywellfit.com/how-to-engage-your-core-the-right-way-4783531#:~:text=You%20should%20be%20able%20to%20continue%20to%20breathe%20when%20you,and%20out%20when%20you%20breathe.

Chair flexing foot pose. (n.d.b.). Tummee. https://www.tummee.com/yoga-poses/chair-flexing-foot-pose

Cobra pose chair. (n.d.c.). Tummee. https://www.tummee.com/yoga-poses/cobra-pose-chair

Davidson, K. (2021, February 9). *Can yoga help aid digestion? 9 poses to try*. Healthline. https://www.healthline.com/nutrition/yoga-posture-for-digestion

Downward facing dog pose variation chair. (n.d.d.). Tummee. https://www.tummee.com/yoga-poses/downward-facing-dog-pose-variation-chair

Eating a balanced diet. (2022, July 29). NHS. https://www.nhs.uk/live-well/eat-well/how-to-eat-a-balanced-diet/eating-a-balanced-diet/

Fowler, S. [fabulous50s]. (2020, August 12). *Lose belly fat sitting down: Ab workout for women over 50!* [Video]. YouTube. https://www.youtube.com/watch?v=tS01JLqO2B8

Freeman, D. [Donna Freeman]. (2017, October 12). *Chair yoga: Core work* [Video]. YouTube. https://www.youtube.com/watch?v=PwyWeeWMx9s

Gate pose on chair. (n.d.e.). Tummee. https://www.tummee.com/yoga-poses/gate-pose-on-chair

Goddess pose on chair arms flow. (n.d.f.). Tummee. https://www.tummee.com/yoga-poses/goddess-pose-on-chair-arms-flow

Gracia, Z. (2023, July). *Chair yoga for stress relief*. BetterMe. https://betterme.world/articles/chair-yoga-for-stress-relief/

Gunnars, K. (2023, November 20). *Intermittent fasting 101—The ultimate beginner's guide*. Healthline. https://www.healthline.com/nutrition/intermittent-fasting-guide

Half moon pose with chair. (n.d.g.). Tummee. https://www.tummee.com/yoga-poses/half-moon-pose-with-chair

Harvard Division of Sleep Medicine. (2021, October 1). *Why sleep matters: Benefits of sleep*. Harvard Medical School. https://sleep.hms.harvard.edu/education-training/public-education/sleep-and-health-education-program/sleep-health-education-41

Hattori, A. [yes2next]. (2022, June 14). *Chair yoga for seniors, beginners* [Video]. YouTube. https://www.youtube.com/watch?v=U_jdXFfegKE

Hattori, A. [yes2next]. (2023, October 17). *Standing chair yoga (beginner friendly): Gentle exercises* [Video]. YouTube. https://www.youtube.com/watch?v=_c5ZMJrwais

Horn, M. [Yoga with Mikah]. (2023, October 22). *Sit-to-stand chair yoga: Build strength and prevent falls!* [Video]. YouTube. https://www.youtube.com/watch?v=R_HXaJRV1i0

How much physical activity do adults need? (2022, June 2). CDC. https://www.cdc.gov/physicalactivity/basics/adults/index.htm#:~:text=Each%20week%20adults%20need%20150,Physical%20Activity%20Guidelines%20for%20Americans.&text=We%20know%20150%20minutes%20of,do%20it%20all%20at%20once.

How to do cat-cow pose in yoga. (2023, October 19). Everyday Yoga. https://www.everydayyoga.com/blogs/guides/how-to-do-cat-cow-pose-in-yoga

Humble warrior pose chair. (n.d.h.). Tummee. https://www.tummee.com/yoga-poses/humble-warrior-pose-chair

Intermittent fasting: What is it, and how does it work? (n.d.). Johns Hopkins Medicine. https://www.hopkinsmedicine.org/health/wellness-and-prevention/intermittent-fasting-what-is-it-and-how-does-it-work

Lauren [SeniorShape Fitness]. (2023, February 8). *Chair exercises for seniors: 10 minute seated workout for legs & lower body* [Video]. YouTube. https://www.youtube.com/watch?v=6nWPnvZDkYo

Leech, J. (2023, April 25). *10 reasons to get more sleep.* Healthline. https://www.healthline.com/nutrition/10-reasons-why-good-sleep-is-important

Lockhart, A. [Wellness By Degrees]. (2021, May 18). *Boat pose adapted to the chair* [Video]. YouTube. https://www.youtube.com/watch?v=7ZUHbNadTOs

Mancella, G. (2020, February 12). *How too much stress can cause weight gain (and what to do about it).* Orlando Health. https://www.orlandohealth.com/content-hub/how-too-much-stress-can-cause-weight-gain-and-what-to-do-about-it#:~:text=in%20excess%20amounts.-,Cortisol%20Can%20Lead%20to%20Weight%20Gain,sweet%2C%20fatty%20and%20salty%20foods.

Marcin, A. (2023, July 24). *How to do chair dips.* Healthline. https://www.healthline.com/health/chair-dips#how-to-do

McManus, K.D. (2018, December 19). *Benefits of a healthy diet—with or without weight loss.* Harvard Health Publishing. https://www.health.harvard.edu/blog/benefits-of-a-healthy-diet-with-or-without-weight-loss-2018121915572

Mishler, A. [Yoga With Adriene]. (2019, February 9). *Yoga for neck, shoulders, upper back: 10-minute yoga quickie* [Video]. YouTube. https://www.youtube.com/watch?v=X3-gKPNyrTA

Mukhwana, J. (2024, February). *12 office chair yoga exercises for when you've had a long day at work.* BetterMe. https://betterme.world/articles/office-chair-yoga/

Munuhe, N. (2023, July). *4 chair workouts for abs you can do at your desk.* BetterMe. https://betterme.world/articles/chair-workouts/

Oakes, K. [Daytona Yoga with Krista]. (2015, October 12). *Standing chair yoga flow* [Video]. YouTube. https://www.youtube.com/watch?v=_n0DzNWjkfc

Payge, K. [Yoga by Kierstie Payge]. (2023, February 5). *Chair yoga for core strength - For seniors* [Video]. YouTube. https://www.youtube.com/watch?v=Dmu7L0jBvKs

Pizer, A. (2022, November 4). *10 chair yoga poses you can do at home*. VeryWell Fit. https://www.verywellfit.com/chair-yoga-poses-3567189

Plank pose ii dolphin arms chair. (n.d.i.). Tummee. https://www.tummee.com/yoga-poses/plank-pose-ii-dolphin-arms-chair

Plank pose with chair. (n.d.j.). Tummee. https://www.tummee.com/yoga-poses/plank-pose-with-chair

Read, T. (2023, April 29). *8 weight-free exercises to tone your arms*. Healthline. https://www.healthline.com/health/fitness-exercise/arm-exercises-no-weights#building-muscle

Revolved chair pose. (n.d.k.). Tummee. https://www.tummee.com/yoga-poses/revolved-chair-pose

Revolved goddess pose chair block hand. (n.d.l.). Tummee. https://www.tummee.com/yoga-poses/revolved-goddess-pose-chair-block-hand

Rose, C. [Carolann Rose Yoga]. (2021, May 11). *30 minute chair yoga: Intermediate chair yoga: Carolann Rose Yoga* [Video]. YouTube. https://www.youtube.com/watch?v=aVB4bM0kas4

Sage marichi pose C chair blocks under foot. (n.d.m.). Tummee. https://www.tummee.com/yoga-poses/sage-marichi-pose-c-chair-blocks-under-foot

Schwartz, L. [Lillah Schwartz]. (2022, November 15). *Purvottanasana reverse plank in chair* [Video]. YouTube. https://www.youtube.com/watch?v=MkN9N06a-Vg

Seated cactus arms chair. (n.d.n.). Tummee. https://www.tummee.com/yoga-poses/seated-cactus-arms-chair

Seated chair one hand behind head elbow knee flow. (n.d.o.). Tummee. https://www.tummee.com/yoga-poses/seated-chair-one-hand-behind-head-elbow-knee-flow

Seated forward fold pose on chair. (n.d.p.). Tummee. https://www.tummee.com/yoga-poses/seated-forward-fold-pose-on-chair

Seated forward fold pose two chairs. (n.d.q.). Tummee. https://www.tummee.com/yoga-poses/seated-forward-fold-pose-two-chairs

Seated palm tree pose side bend flow chair. (n.d.r.). Tummee. https://www.tummee.com/yoga-poses/seated-palm-tree-pose-side-bend-flow-chair

Sitting twist pose on chair hand on floor. (n.d.s.). Tummee. https://www.tummee.com/yoga-poses/sitting-twist-pose-on-chair-hand-on-floor

Standing lateral side bend flexion chair. (n.d.t.). Tummee. https://www.tummee.com/yoga-poses/standing-lateral-side-bend-flexion-chair

Standing table top pose hands chair torso circles. (n.d.u.). Tummee. https://www.tummee.com/yoga-poses/standing-table-top-pose-hands-chair-torso-circles

Sun breaths. (n.d.v.). Tummee. https://www.tummee.com/yoga-poses/sun-breaths

Tavino, C.C. [Candace Cabrera Tavino]. (2017, June 22). *10 minute chair yoga for neck, shoulders, back and chest* [Video]. YouTube. https://www.youtube.com/watch?v=oGjdyn4JZhM

Triangle pose chair against wall. (n.d.w.). Tummee. https://www.tummee.com/yoga-poses/triangle-pose-chair-against-wall

10 reasons why hydration is important. (2024, January 16). National Council on Aging. https://www.ncoa.org/article/10-reasons-why-hydration-is-important

Upward facing dog pose with chair. (n.d.x.). Tummee. https://www.tummee.com/yoga-poses/upward-facing-dog-pose-with-chair

Water and Healthier Drinks. (2022, June 6). CDC. https://www.cdc.gov/healthyweight/healthy_eating/water-and-healthier-drinks.html

Weber, B. (2023, August 29). *Stress and weight gain: The connection and how to manage it*. Medical News Today. https://www.medicalnewstoday.com/articles/stress-and-weight-gain#how-it-happens

YJ Editors. (2023, January 1). *High lunge, crescent variation*. Yoga Journal. https://www.y4c.org/news/2018/4/12/variations-of-chair-and-crescent-lunge

Image References

Braun, N. (2022). *A group of people dancing* [Image]. Unsplash. https://unsplash.com/photos/a-group-of-people-dancing-dUhK08-mBn8

Lark, B. (2017). *White ceramic plate beside gray steel spoon* [Image]. Unsplash. https://unsplash.com/photos/white-ceramic-plate-beside-gray-steel-spoon-nBtmglfYoHU

Prophsee Journals. (2019). *Life is your creation card* [Image]. Unsplash. https://unsplash.com/photos/life-is-your-creation-card-sFTMwH2Tvec

Rae, S. (2017). *Brown dried leaves on sand* [Image]. Unsplash. https://unsplash.com/photos/brown-dried-leaves-on-sand-geM5lzDj4Iw

Made in the USA
Middletown, DE
06 September 2024

60478939R00091